Avoid Dialysis

10 Step Diet Plan for Healthier Kidneys

Nina Kolbe RD CSR LD
Nina@kidneyhealthgourmet.com

Other books by this author

Kidney Health Gourmet Diet Guide and Cookbook

A recommended companion book to the 10 Step Diet Plan: Kidney Health Gourmet; Diet Guide and Cookbook. A collection of recipes for People Not on Dialysis. Not just kidney friendly recipes; included is a beverage guide, eating out guide, frozen meal comparison, milk comparison even a guide to which lettuce is lowest in potassium.

See order form in back of this book.

First published in 2009
Revised and updated 2011
Revised and updated 2014

Contents

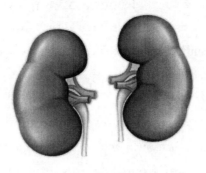

CHAPTER 1

THE BASICS

Can I really stop the decline in kidney function? Absolutely, yes! The top two reasons for failing kidneys are diabetes and hypertension. Both can be managed and prevent damage to the kidneys. There are also other reasons for decreased kidney function. In my practice I have dozens of success stories and you can be one of them too!

Let me first tell you about how this book came to be written and my background. I am a renal dietitian, which means I have chosen to specialize my practice with patients who have kidney disease. I am a Board Certified Specialist in Renal Nutrition, but enough about me. For the past 15 years I have worked with dialysis patients. To dispel some myths you may have heard, these people can lead full lives. Many of them work, travel, attend social functions and feel good most of the time. Over the years I have had many conversations with these patients, many did not really know what caused their kidneys to fail. Many did know, and wished they could turn back the clock and make different choices that would have salvaged their kidneys.

Today we have tests that allow us to identify very early any changes in kidney function. Once we know that a person has some diminished kidney function there is so much that can be done. If some of my patients were identified earlier and had been counseled, their lives would have turned out much differently.

I felt drawn to write this book to give all of you the opportunity to change the outcome and preserve your kidneys. I want to empower you with information and lead you to make good choices and which will have positive outcomes to your health. I don't profess to have the same knowledge as your Nephrologist and I hope you are seeing one. I want to empower you with knowledge about your disease, diet, lab testing, and medications. With this knowledge. You can ask your health care team the right questions and make improvements to your lifestyle. I have provided you with a 10 steps plan to improve your health. If you follow these 10 steps you are sure to improve the course of your kidney disease.

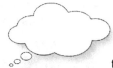 Let me tell you about some of my patients that I see in my CKD practice. These patients have been diagnosed with decreased kidney function but are not on dialysis.

Jane Doe a 40-year-old type 2 diabetic. She had a large quantity of protein in her urine, which is evidence of impaired kidney function or difficult-to-control hypertension.

At 38 ml/min, her glomerular filtration rate, or GFR—a measure of kidney function—suggested she already had moderate kidney damage. She had a large amount of protein in her urine, poorly controlled hypertension, and poorly controlled blood sugar.

Her disease was in stage 3 of CKD. When she learned that she may be heading toward dialysis, it was a shock and it motivated her to make many changes.

Jane cut sodium in her diet, started an exercise plan, and lost weight, which helped improve her blood pressure and blood glucose. She monitored her blood sugar more carefully than before, and worked closely with me and her physicians to maintain good glycemic control.

Three years have passed and this patient is doing quite well. Her blood pressure is under control and excellent blood sugar levels with an HgA1c of 6.5. (See diabetic chapter)

John Doe is a 52-year-old male diagnosed with high blood pressure. He was so alarmed at being diagnosed with CKD stage 4 that he became a vegetarian. This was a red meat and potato kind of guy but the shock of his diagnosis caused him to take drastic action. He became a vegetarian with occasional binges on cheeseburgers. He lost 30 lbs., maintained his blood pressure less than 120/80 and improved his kidney function to stage 3 CKD.

I am not advocating a vegetarian life style, although if it suits you then why not. I am encouraging you not to feel hopeless, but empowered to make necessary health changes and take charge of your destiny.

Every step you take to improve you health such as diet, controlling your blood pressure, starting an exercise program will only improve your health and the health of your kidneys.

Take charge of your health and your destiny! Let's start with the basics such as ...

What functions do the kidneys perform

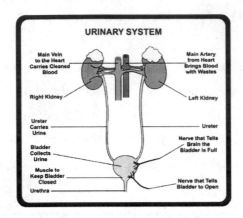

URINARY SYSTEM

Main Vein to the Heart Carries Cleaned Blood

Main Artery from Heart Brings Blood with Wastes

Right Kidney

Left Kidney

Ureter Carries Urine

Ureter

Nerve that Tells Brain the Bladder is Full

Bladder Collects Urine

Muscle to Keep Bladder Closed

Nerve that Tells Bladder to Open

Urethra

The kidneys are bean-shaped organs, each about the size of a fist. They are located near the middle of the back, just below the rib cage, one on each side of the spine. The kidneys are sophisticated reprocessing machines. Every day, a person's kidneys process about 200 quarts of blood to sift out about 2 quarts of waste products and extra water. The wastes and extra water become urine, which flows to the bladder through tubes called ureters. The bladder stores urine until releasing it through urination.

Wastes in the blood come from the normal breakdown of active tissues, such as muscles, and from food. The body uses food for energy and self-repairs. After the body has taken what it needs from food, wastes are sent to the blood. And the kidneys remove them through urine. If the kidneys did not remove them, these wastes would build up in the blood and damage the body.

The actual removal of wastes occurs in tiny units inside the kidneys called nephrons. Each kidney has about a million nephrons. In the nephron, a glomerulus—which is a tiny blood vessel, or capillary—intertwines with a tiny urine- collecting tube called a tubule. The glomerulus acts as a filtering unit, or sieve, and keeps normal proteins and cells in the bloodstream, allowing extra fluid and wastes to pass through. A complicated chemical exchange takes place, as waste materials and water leave the blood and enter the urinary system.

At first, the tubules receive a combination of waste materials and chemicals the body can still use. The kidneys measure out chemicals like sodium, phosphorus, and potassium and release them back to the blood to return to the body. In this way, the kidneys regulate the body's level of these substances. The right balance is necessary for life.

In addition to removing wastes, the kidneys make three important hormones:

- Erythropoietin, or EPO, which stimulates the bone marrow to make red blood cells

- Renin, which regulates blood pressure

- Calcitriol, the active form of vitamin D, which helps maintain calcium for bones and for normal chemical balance in the body

What is renal function?

The word "renal" refers to the kidneys. The terms "renal function" and "kidney function" mean the same thing.

Health professionals use the term "renal function" to mean how efficiently the kidneys filter blood. People with two healthy kidneys have 100 percent of their kidney function. Small or mild declines in kidney function—as much as 30 to 40 percent—would rarely be noticeable.

Kidney function is now calculated using a blood sample and a formula to find the estimated glomerular filtration rate (eGFR). The eGFR corresponds to the percent of kidney function. Some people are born with only one kidney but can still lead normal, healthy lives.

For many people with reduced kidney function, kidney disease may be present it may further cause decline in kidney function. Progressive health problems occur when people have less than 25 percent of their kidney function. When kidney function drops below 5 percent, a person may need some renal replacement therapy—either blood-cleansing treatments called dialysis or a kidney transplant.

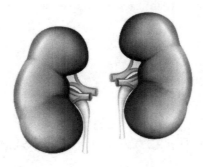

CHAPTER TWO

CAUSES OF DECREASE IN KIDNEY FUNCTION

Chronic kidney disease is slow to develop and progress. The disease destroys the nephrons of the kidney slowly and silently. Only after years or even decades will the damage become apparent. Most kidney diseases attack both kidneys simultaneously. This slow type of kidney disease is known as chronic kidney disease.

The two most common causes of kidney disease are diabetes and high blood pressure. People with a family history of any kind of kidney problem are at risk for kidney disease.

Diabetic Kidney Disease

Diabetes is a disease that keeps the body from managing glucose, a form of sugar. If too much glucose stays in the blood instead of being used by the cells, it can have a negative impact. Damage to the nephrons from excess glucose in the blood is called diabetic kidney disease. Keeping blood glucose levels at a physiologic level can delay or prevent diabetic kidney disease

High Blood Pressure

High blood pressure can damage the small blood vessels in the kidneys. The damaged vessels cannot filter wastes from the blood adequately. High blood pressure can lead to kidney disease. It can also be a sign that the kidneys are already impaired. The only way to know whether a person's blood pressure is high is to have a health professional measure it with a blood pressure cuff. The result is expressed as two numbers. The top number, which is called the systolic pressure, represents the pressure in the blood vessels when the heart is beating. The bottom number, which is called the diastolic pressure, shows the pressure when the heart is resting between beats. A person's blood pressure is considered normal if it stays below 120/80, stated as 120 over 80. The National Heart Lung and Blood Institute (NHLBI) recommends that people with kidney disease use whatever therapy is necessary, including lifestyle changes and medicines, to keep their blood pressure below 130/80.

Glomerular Diseases and Nephrotic Syndrome

Several types of kidney disease are grouped together under this category, including autoimmune diseases, infection- related diseases, and sclerotic diseases. As the name indicates, glomerular diseases attack the tiny blood vessels, or glomeruli, within the kidney.

Membranous nephropathy (MN)

A type of kidney disease in which the small blood vessels in the kidney that filter wastes become thick and inflamed. MN can cause nephrotic syndrome, which can lead to long-term kidney damage if left untreated.

Focal segmental glomerulosclerosis (FSGS)

A type of kidney disease in which scar tissue forms on the glomeruli (small blood vessels in the kidney that filter wastes).

Minimal change disease (MCD)

A type of kidney disease in which the small blood vessels in the kidney that filter wastes are damaged, but the effects are not visible under a regular microscope. Instead, the damage can only be seen through an electron microscope.

Membranoproliferative glomerulonephritis (MPGN)

A type of kidney disease in which inflammation and abnormal changes occur in kidney cells. MPGN can cause nephrotic syndrome.

IgA nephropathy (IgA)

A type of kidney disease that causes inflammation in the small blood vessels of the kidney. This keeps them from effectively filtering waste products and excess water from the bloodstream. It is most often associated with other diseases, including diabetes, malaria, hepatitis, or systemic lupus erythematous.

Systemic lupus erythematous (SLE)

An autoimmune disease, which means that the immune system mistakes the bodies own tissues as foreign invaders and attacks them. Some people with lupus suffer only minor inconvenience. Others may have major organs affected.

Lupus affects people of African, Asian, or Native American descent two to three times as often as it affects whites. Nine out of 10 people with lupus are women. The disease usually strikes between age 15 and 44, although it can occur in older individuals.

SLE may inflame and/or damage the connective tissue in the joints, muscles, and skin, along with the membranes surrounding or within the lungs, heart, kidneys, and brain. SLE can also cause kidney disease called Lupus Nephritis. Up to 60% of lupus patients will develop lupus nephritis. When the kidneys are inflamed, they can't function normally and can leak protein. If not controlled, lupus nephritis can lead to kidney failure.

The first sign of a glomerular disease is often proteinuria, which is too much protein in the urine. Another common sign is hematuria, which is blood in the urine. Some people may have both proteinuria and hematuria. Glomerular diseases can slowly destroy kidney function. Blood pressure control is important with any kidney disease. Glomerular diseases are usually diagnosed with a biopsy—a procedure that involves taking a piece of kidney tissue for examination under a microscope. Treatments for glomerular diseases may include immunosuppressive drugs or steroids to reduce inflammation and proteinuria, depending on the specific disease. See last chapter for new treatments using Acthar.

Inherited and Congenital Kidney Diseases

Some kidney diseases result from hereditary factors. Polycystic kidney disease (PKD), for example, is a genetic disorder in which many cysts grow in the kidneys. PKD cysts can slowly replace much of the mass of the kidneys, reducing kidney function and leading to kidney failure.

In early stages of the disease, the cysts enlarge the kidney and interfere with kidney function, resulting in chronic high blood pressure and kidney infections. The cysts may cause the kidneys to increase production of erythropoietin (the hormone that stimulates production of red blood cells) resulting in too many red blood cells, rather than the expected anemia of chronic kidney disease.

PKD comes in two forms. Autosomal Dominant Polycystic Kidney Disease (ADPKD) is the most common, affecting 1-in-400 to 1-in-500 adults. Autosomal Recessive Polycystic Kidney Disease (ARPKD) is far less common, affecting 1-in-10, 000 at a far younger age, including newborns, infants and children.

Other Causes of
Kidney Disease Immune diseases

Lupus. A chronic inflammatory disease, lupus can affect many parts of your body, including your skin, joints, kidneys, blood cells, heart and lungs.

Good pasture's syndrome. A rare immune lung disorder that may mimic pneumonia, Good pasture's syndrome causes bleeding (hemorrhage) into your lungs as well as glomerulonephritis.

Infections

Post-streptococcal glomerulonephritis. Glomerulonephritis may develop after a strep infection in your throat or, rarely, on your skin (impetigo). Post-infectious glomerulonephritis is becoming less common in the United States, most likely because of rapid and complete antibiotic treatment of most streptococcal infections.

Viral infections. Among the viral infections that may trigger glomerulonephritis are the human immunodeficiency virus (HIV), which causes AIDS, and the hepatitis B and hepatitis C viruses, which primarily affect the liver.

Poisons and trauma, such as a direct and forceful blow to the kidneys, can lead to kidney disease.

Some over-the-counter medicines can be poisonous to the kidneys if taken regularly over a long period of time. Anyone who takes painkillers regularly should check with a doctor to make sure the kidneys are not at risk.

Kidney Stones

Frequent passing of kidney stones over the years can cause damage to the kidneys. (See kidney stone chapter for diet and treatment).

Acute Kidney Injury

Some kidney problems happen quickly, such as when an accident injures the kidneys. Losing a lot of blood can cause sudden kidney failure. Some drugs or poisons can make the kidneys stop working. These sudden drops in kidney function are called acute kidney injury (AKI). Some doctors may also refer to this condition as acute renal failure (ARF). AKI may lead to permanent loss of kidney function. But if the kidneys are not seriously damaged, acute kidney disease may be reversed. However, there is research that shows that prior history of AKI may be make a future diagnosis of CKD more likely. A person who has had an AKI/AKF episode should be especially careful to take care of their kidneys to prevent CKD in the future.

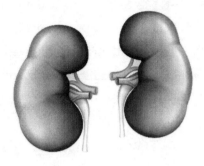

CHAPTER 3

WHAT ARE THE
STAGES OF KIDNEY DISEASE

Stage 1. A person's glomerular filtration rate (eGFR) is the best indicator of how well the kidneys are working. An eGFR of 90 or above is considered normal. A person whose eGFR stays below 60 for 3 months or longer has chronic kidney disease. As kidney function declines, the risk of complications rises.

Stage 2 GFR 60-89. Mildly low GFR a, great opportunity to find out what is causing the strain on the kidney and follow your Nephrologist's advice along with my recommendations to get your kidney back to their full health.

Stage 3 Moderate decrease in eGFR (30 to 59). At this stage of CKD, hormones and minerals can be thrown out of balance, leading to anemia and weaker bones. This is an excellent opportunity to have heard the warning, at this stage diet, blood pressure, glycemic control, exercise, seeing a Nephrologist can help prevent or treat further complications and stabilize your disease.

Stage 4 Severe reduction in eGFR (15 to 29). This patient should continue following the treatment for complications of CKD. I have seen patients in stage 4, who were extremely committed to their health. They changed their diet, followed their Nephrologist's advice, started an exercise plan, lost weight, and controlled their blood pressure and blood glucose. Their careful attention to their health kept them at this stage without requiring dialysis.

Kidney failure (eGFR less than 15). When the kidneys are not filtering sufficiently, removal of fluid is impaired; dialysis or a kidney transplant may be indicated.

In addition to tracking eGFR, blood tests can show when substances in the blood are out of balance. If phosphorus or potassium levels start to climb, a blood test will prompt the health care provider to address these issues before they permanently affect the patient's health.

What are the signs of chronic kidney disease (CKD)?

People in the early stages of CKD may have very few symptoms or none at all.

As kidney disease progresses, some symptoms may appear:

- change in urination pattern
- feeling tired
- loss of appetite, nausea or vomiting
- swollen hands or feet
- feeling itchy or numb
- drowsiness or loss of concentration

- darkened skin
- muscle cramps

What medical tests detect kidney disease?

Because a person can have kidney disease without any symptoms, a doctor may first detect the condition through routine blood and urine tests. Three tests screen for kidney disease: a blood pressure measurement, a spot check for protein or albumin in the urine, and a calculation of glomerular filtration rate (GFR) based on a serum creatinine measurement. Measuring urea nitrogen in the blood provides additional information.

Microalbuminuria and Proteinuria

Healthy kidneys take wastes out of the blood but leave protein behind. Impaired kidneys may fail to separate a blood protein called albumin from the wastes. At first, only small amount of albumin may leak into the urine, a condition known as microalbuminuria, a sign of deteriorating kidney function. As kidney function declines, the amount of albumin and other proteins in the urine increases, and the condition is called proteinuria. A doctor may test for protein using a dipstick in a small sample of a person's urine taken in the doctor's office. The color of the dipstick indicates the presence or absence of proteinuria.

A more sensitive test for protein or albumin in the urine involves laboratory measurement and calculation of the protein-to-creatinine or albumin-to-creatinine ratio.

Creatinine is a waste product in the blood created by the normal breakdown of muscle cells during activity. Healthy kidneys take creatinine out of the blood and put it into the urine to leave the body. When the kidneys are not working well, creatinine builds up in the blood.

The albumin-to-creatinine measurement should be used to detect kidney disease in people at high risk, especially those with diabetes or high blood pressure. If a person's first laboratory test shows high levels of protein, another test should be done 1 to 2 weeks later. If the second test also shows high levels of protein, the person has persistent proteinuria and should have additional tests to evaluate kidney function.

Urine Creatinine: This test estimates the concentration of your urine and helps to give an accurate protein result. Protein-to-Creatinine Ratio: This estimates the amount of protein you excrete in your urine in a day and avoids the need to collect a 24-hour sample of your urine.

Glomerular Filtration Rate (GFR) Based on Creatinine Measurement

GFR is a calculation of how efficiently the kidneys are filtering wastes from the blood. A traditional GFR calculation requires an injection into the bloodstream of a substance that is later measured in a 24-hour urine collection. Recently, scientists found they could calculate GFR without an injection or urine collection. The new calculation—the eGFR—requires only a measurement of the creatinine in a blood sample.

In a laboratory, a person's blood is tested to see how many milligrams of creatinine are in one deciliter of blood (mg/dL). Creatinine levels in the blood can vary, and each laboratory has its own normal range, usually 0.6 to 1.2 mg/dL. A person whose creatinine level is only slightly above this range will probably not feel sick, but the elevation is a sign that the kidneys are not working at full strength. One formula for estimating kidney function equates a creatinine level of 1.7 mg/dL for most men and 1.4 mg/dL for most women to 50 percent of normal kidney function. Because creatinine values are so variable and can be affected by diet, a GFR calculation is more accurate for determining whether a person has reduced kidney function.

The eGFR calculation uses the patient's creatinine measurement along with age and values assigned for sex and race. Some medical laboratories may make the eGFR calculation when a creatinine value is measured and include it on the lab report. The National Kidney Foundation has determined different stages of CKD based on the value of the eGFR. Dialysis or transplantation is needed when the eGFR is less than 15 milliliters per minute (mL/min).

Blood Urea Nitrogen (BUN)

Blood carries protein to cells throughout the body. After the cells use the protein, the remaining waste product is returned to the blood as urea, a compound that contains nitrogen. Healthy kidneys take urea out of the blood and excrete it in the urine. If a person's kidneys are not working well, some of the urea may stay in the blood.

A deciliter of normal blood contains 7 to 20 milligrams of urea. If a person's BUN is more than 20 mg/dL, the kidneys may not be working at full strength. Other possible causes of an elevated BUN include dehydration and heart failure.

Phosphorus: Goal 2.7-4.6 a high phosphorus level can lead to weak bones. If your level is too high, your doctor may ask you to reduce your intake of foods that are high in phosphorus, especially processed food. If dietary changes are inadequate to lower your phosphorus level, then a type of medication called a phosphate binder may be suggested. To be taken with meals and snacks.

Potassium: Goal 3.5-5.2 Potassium is a mineral in your blood that helps your heart and muscles work properly. A potassium level that is too high or too low may weaken muscles and change your heartbeat. Whether you need to change the amount of high- potassium foods in your diet depends on your stage of kidney disease. Please note that constipation can give you a falsely high reading on your blood test. Make sure that you inform your doctor of this or reschedule your test if have have not had a bowel movement for 2 days.

Calcium: Goal 8.4-9.5 Calcium is a mineral that is important for strong bones. To help balance the amount of calcium in your blood, your doctor may ask you to take calcium supplements and a special prescription form of vitamin D. Take only the supplements and medications recommended by your doctor. Make sure you share with your physician all supplements, antacids and vitamins you are taking.

Parathyroid Hormone (PTH): High levels of parathyroid hormone (PTH) may result from a poor balance of calcium and phosphorus in your body. This can cause bone disease. Ask your doctor if your PTH level is in the right range. Your doctor may order a special prescription form of vitamin D to help lower your PTH. Caution: Do not take over-the-counter vitamin D or calcium unless ordered by your doctor.

Serum Albumin: Goal 4.0 or greater. Albumin is a protein made by the liver from the protein eat. A low level of albumin in your blood may be caused by not consuming adequate protein or calories from your diet. A low level of albumin may lead to health problems such as compromised immune system manifested by difficulty fighting off infections. It is often a balancing act to make sure a person is getting the right amount of protein but just enough. See protein calculation to determine your ideal protein intake.

TSAT and Serum Ferritin: Your TSAT and serum ferritin are measures of iron in your body. Your TSAT should be above 20 percent and your serum ferritin should be above 100. This will help you build red blood cells. Your doctor may recommend iron supplements when needed to reach your target levels. If the iron levels drop severely an iron infusion in a doctor's office may be indicated.

Hemoglobin: Goal 11-12. Hemoglobin is the part of red blood cells that carries oxygen from your lungs to all parts of your body. Your hemoglobin level tells your doctor if you have anemia, which makes you feel tired and have little energy. If you have anemia, you may need treatment with iron supplements and a hormone called erythropoietin (EPO). The goal of anemia treatment is to reach and maintain a hemoglobin level of at least 11 to 12.

Hematocrit: Goal 33-36%. Your hematocrit is a measure of the red blood cells your body is making. A low hematocrit can mean you have anemia and need treatment with iron and EPO. You will feel less tired and have more energy when your hematocrit reaches at least 33 to 36 percent.

Total Cholesterol: Goal under 200. Cholesterol is a fat-like substance found in your blood. A high cholesterol level may increase your chance of having heart and circulation problems. For many patients, a good level for total cholesterol is below 200. If your cholesterol level is too high, your doctor may ask you to make some changes in your diet and increase your activity level. In some cases, medications are also used.

HDL Cholesterol: Goal above 40. HDL cholesterol is a type of "good" cholesterol that protects your heart.

LDL Cholesterol: Goal under 100. LDL cholesterol is a type of "bad" cholesterol. A high LDL level may increase your chance of having heart and circulation problems. If your LDL level is too high, your doctor may ask you to make some changes in your diet and increase your activity level.

Triglyceride: Goal under 150. Triglyceride is a type of fat found in your blood. A high triglyceride level along with high levels of total and LDL cholesterol may increase your chance of heart and circulation problems.

Additional Tests for Kidney Disease

If blood and urine tests indicate reduced kidney function, a doctor may recommend additional tests to help identify the cause of the problem.

Kidney imaging. Methods of kidney imaging—taking pictures of the kidneys—include ultrasound, computerized tomography (CT) scan, and magnetic resonance imaging (MRI). These tools are most helpful in finding unusual growths or blockages to the flow of urine.

Kidney biopsy. A doctor may want to examine a tiny piece of kidney tissue with a microscope. To obtain this tissue sample, the doctor will perform a kidney biopsy—a hospital procedure in which the doctor inserts a needle through the patient's skin into the back of the kidney. The needle retrieves a strand of tissue less than an inch long.

For the procedure, the patient lies facedown on a table and receives a local anesthetic to numb the skin. The sample tissue will help the doctor identify problems at the cellular level.

There are other tests that I want you to become familiar with and keep a detailed record for yourself. I have provided a tool for you to keep track of the tests which will help you follow you kidney status as well as be aware of necessary dietary changes.

Lab tracking grid

Test	What it means	Ckd values	Date	Date	Date	Date
Creatinine	Waste product of protein					
BUN	Measure of waste					
GFR	Estimate of kidney function					
Potassium	Mineral in the blood	3.5-5.2				
Phosphorus	Mineral in the blood	2.7-4.6				
Calcium	Mineral inthe blood	8.4-9.5				
Hgb	Red bloodcells	11-14				
Glucose	Measure of blood sugar	Fast-ing <100				
HgA1c	Blood sugar past 3 months	Goal 6.5-7.0				
Cholesterol	Fat like substance	Goal <200				

HDL chol	Good cholesterol	
LDL chol	Bad cholesterol	Goal <100
Triglycerides	Blood fat	Goal <150
Vit D	Level in the blood	Goal >30
Albumin	Measure of good nutrition	Goal >4.0

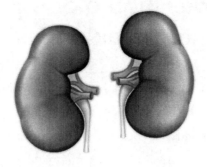

CHAPTER 4

STEP 1 CONTROL YOUR BLOOD PRESSURE

Normal Blood Pressure

A typical blood pressure reading is 120/80.

What is high blood pressure?

High blood pressure also called hypertension can result from too much fluid in normal blood vessels or from normal fluid in narrow blood vessels. Blood pressure measures the force of blood against the walls of your blood vessels. Blood pressure that remains high over time is called hypertension. Extra fluid in your body increases the amount of fluid in your blood vessels and makes your blood pressure higher. Narrow or clogged blood vessels also raise your blood pressure. If you have high blood pressure, see your doctor regularly.

How does high blood pressure hurt my kidneys?

High blood pressure makes your heart work harder and, over time, can damage blood vessels throughout your body. If the blood vessels in your kidneys are damaged, they may stop removing wastes and extra fluid from your body. The extra fluid in your blood vessels may then raise blood pressure even more. It's a dangerous cycle.

How will I know whether I have high blood pressure?

Most people with high blood pressure have no symptoms. The only way to know whether your blood pressure is high is to have a health professional measure it with a blood pressure cuff. The result is expressed as two numbers. The top number, which is called the systolic pressure, represents the pressure when your heart is beating. The bottom number, which is called the diastolic pressure, shows the pressure when your heart is resting between beats. Your blood pressure is considered normal if it stays below 120/80 (expressed as "120 over 80"). People with a systolic blood pressure of 120 to 139 or a diastolic blood pressure of 80 to 89 are considered pre-hypertensive and should adopt health-promoting lifestyle changes to prevent diseases of the heart and blood vessels. If your systolic blood pressure is consistently 140 or higher or your diastolic pressure is 90 or higher, you have high blood pressure and should talk with your doctor about the best ways to lower it.

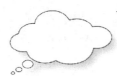 When I first meet with a new patient I always ask if they have high blood pressure. Most people say no and after much probing they reveal that "yes, they did have it but they don't have it anymore because they take

28

medications to control it". I want to add that just because you take medications you can't assume that you are well controlled. *The take away for you is know what your blood pressure is and take all the steps necessary to make sure you are in range. You are about to learn how.*

Kidney damage, like hypertension, can be unnoticeable and detected only through medical tests. Blood tests will show whether your kidneys are removing wastes efficiently.

How can I prevent high blood pressure from damaging my kidneys?

If you have kidney damage, you should keep your blood pressure below 130/80. The National Heart, Lung, and Blood Institute (NHLBI), one of the National Institutes of Health (NIH), recommends that people with kidney disease use whatever therapy is necessary, including lifestyle changes and medicines, to keep their blood pressure below 130/80.

How can I control my blood pressure?

NHLBI has found that five lifestyle changes can help control blood pressure:

Maintain your weight at a level close to normal. Choose fruits, vegetables, grains, and low-fat dairy foods.

Limit your daily sodium (salt) intake to 2,000 milligrams or lower if you already have high blood pressure. Read nutrition labels on packaged foods to learn how much sodium is in one serving. Make sure you read the label carefully. For example a label of 1 can of soup may say that it contains 800 mg per serving. Upon closer scrutiny you may see that there are actually 2 servings in a can. Since most people will eat the entire can, they are likely to consume 1600 mg of sodium from that soup. This is almost the entire days worth of sodium. Keeping a sodium diary to track sodium intake may be helpful.

Get plenty of exercise, which means at least 30 minutes of moderate activity, such as walking every day.

Avoid consuming too much alcohol. Men should limit consumption to two drinks (two 12-ounce servings of beer or two 5-ounce servings of wine or two 1.5-ounce servings of "hard" liquor) a day. Women should have no more than a single serving on a given day.

A doctor may prescribe blood pressure medication. ACE inhibitors and ARBs have been found to protect the kidneys even more than other medicines that lower blood pressure to similar levels. The National Heart, Lung, and Blood Institute (NHLBI), one of the National Institutes of Health, recommends that people with diabetes or reduced kidney function keep their blood pressure below 130/80.

ACE Inhibitors

What are ACE inhibitors, and how do they work? Angiotensin II is a very potent chemical that causes the muscles surrounding blood vessels to contract, thereby narrowing the vessels. The narrowing of the vessels increases the pressure within the vessels causing high blood pressure (hypertension). Angiotensin II is formed from angiotensin I in the blood by the enzyme angiotensin-converting enzyme (ACE). ACE inhibitors are medications that slow (inhibit) the activity of the enzyme ACE, which decreases the production of angiotensin II. As a result, the blood vessels enlarge or dilate, and blood pressure is reduced. This lower blood pressure makes it easier for the heart to pump blood and can improve the function of a failing heart. In addition, the progression of kidney disease due to high blood pressure or diabetes is slowed. The down side of ACE inhibitors is that they may cause the body to retain potassium. Since it is beneficial to take these medications, extra care should be taken to lower dietary potassium if you note that your potassium level is rising. Use the lab grid provided to track your potassium levels.

What are some examples of ACE inhibitors

The following is a list of the ACE inhibitors that are available in the United States:

benazepril (Lotensin)

captopril (Capoten)

enalapril (Vasotec)

fosinopril (Monopril)

lisinopril (Prinivil, Zestril)

moexipril (Univasc)

perindopril (Aceon)

quinapril (Accupril)

ramipril (Altace)

trandolapril (Mavik)

Angiotensin II Receptor Blockers (ARB)

What are angiotensin receptor blockers and how do they work?

Angiotensin II is a very potent chemical that causes the muscles surrounding the blood vessels to contract, which thereby narrows the blood vessels. This narrowing increases the pressure within the vessels and can cause high blood pressure. Angiotensin receptor blockers (ARBs) are medications that block the action of angiotensin II. As a result, the blood vessels dilate and the blood pressure is reduced. The lower blood pressure makes it easier for the heart to pump blood and can improve heart failure. In addition, the progression of kidney disease due to high blood pressure or diabetes is slowed.

For what conditions are ARBs used?

ARBs are used for controlling high blood pressure, treating heart failure, and preventing kidney failure in people with diabetes or high blood pressure. Since these medications have effects that are similar to those of ACE Inhibitors they are often used when patients cannot tolerate an ACE inhibitor.

The following is a list of currently available ARBs:

candesartan (Atacand)

eprosartan Tevetan

irbesartan (Avapro)

telmisartan (Mycardis)

valsartan (Diovan)

losartan (Cozaar)

Sodium

Salt in the diet

Many people think of salt and sodium as being the same thing, but they are not. Table salt is 40 percent sodium and 60 percent chloride. It is the sodium portion of salt that is important to people concerned about high blood pressure. Keep in mind some sodium is naturally present in most foods.

Quick Facts...

- Sodium is one factor in the development of high blood pressure.

- Sodium is made up of salt; table salt is 40 percent sodium and 60 percent chloride.

- Most foods contain some sodium because it is naturally present.

- The recommended level of sodium intake is 2,000 mg per day.

Sodium is a part of everyone's diet, but how much is too much? Under ideal conditions, the minimum sodium requirement is about 1,500 milligrams (mg) of sodium each day. This is les than 1 teaspoon of table salt. The maximum recommended level of sodium intake is 2,000 mg per day. On average, American men consume between 3000 and 4,500 mg of sodium per day, while women consume between 2,5300 and 3,200 mg (due to their lower calorie intake, not because of restricting sodium).

Sodium intake is one factor involved in the development of high blood pressure, otherwise known as hypertension.

Hypertension tends to develop as people age. Some individuals are "salt sensitive," so reducing intake of sodium helps to reduce blood pressure levels. A high intake of sodium early in life might weaken genetic defenses against developing high blood pressure. Experts recommend not to wait and see if you develop hypertension, but to reduce sodium intake while blood pressure is still normal. This may decrease your risk of developing hypertension.

Where is Sodium Found?

Most of the sodium in processed foods is added to preserve or flavor them. Salt is the major source of this sodium. Salt is added to most canned and some frozen vegetables, smoked and cured meats, pickles and sauerkraut. It is used in most cheeses, sauces, soups, salad dressings and many breakfast cereals. It is also found in many other ingredients used in food processing.

Watch out for commercially prepared condiments, sauces and seasonings when preparing and serving foods for you and your family. Many, like those in Table 1, are high in sodium.

The link between salt and sodium may be a little hard to understand at first. If you remember that one-teaspoon of salt provides 2,000 milligrams of sodium, however, you can estimate the amount of sodium that you add to foods during cooking and preparation, or even at the tables

Where does sodium come from in your diet?

5% added while cooking

6% added while eating

12% from natural soures

77% from processed and prepared foods

Salt-Sodium Conversions

- $1/4$ tsp. salt = 500 mg sodium

- ½ tsp. salt = 1,000 mg sodium

- ¾ tsp. salt = 1,500 mg sodium

- 1 tsp. salt = 2,000 mg sodium

Table 1: Sodium comparisons.			
Little sodium	**Low sodium**	**More sodium**	**High sodium**
Apple, 2 mg	**Applesauce,** 1 c., 6 mg	**Apple pie,** ⅛, frozen, 208 mg	**Apple pie**, 1, fast food, 400 mg
Low sodium bread, 1 slice, 7 mg	**Bread, white** 1 slice, 114 mg	**Pound cake,** 1 slice, 171 mg	**English muffin,** whole, 203 mg
Vegetable oil, 1 tbsp., 0 mg	**Butter**, 1 tbsp., unsalted, 2 mg	**Butter**, 1 tbsp., salted, 116 mg	**Margarine,** 1 tbsp., 140 mg
Chicken, ½ breast, 69 mg	**Chicken pie,** 1, frozen, 997 mg	**Chicken noodle soup**, 1 c., 1,107 mg	**Chicken dinner** Fast food, 2,443 mg
Fresh corn, 1ear, 1 mg	**Frozen corn,** 1 c., 7 mg	**Corn flakes,** 1 c., 256 mg	**Canned corn**, 1 c., 243 mg, 384 mg
Cucumber, 7 slices, 2 mg	**Sweet pickle,** 1, 128 mg	**Cucumber w/ salad w dressing,** 234 mg	**Dill pickle**, 1, 928 mg

Table 1: Sodium comparisons.			
Little sodium	**Low sodium**	**More sodium**	**High sodium**
Pork, fresh 3 oz., 59 mg	**Bacon**, 4 slices, 548 mg	**Frankfurter**, 1, 639 mg	**Ham**, 3 oz., 1,114 mg
Lemon, 1, 1 mg	**Catsup**, 1 tbsp., 156 mg	**Soy sauce**, 1 tbsp., 1,02mg	**Salt**, 1 tsp., 1, 938 mg
Potato, 1, 5 mg	**Potato chips**, 10, 200 mg	**Mashed potatoes**, instant, 1c, 485 mg	Potato salad, ½ cup, 625 mg
Plain yogurt, 1 c., 105 mg	**Milk**, 1 c., 122 mg	**Buttermilk**, 1 c., 257 mg	**Choc. Pudding**, ½ c instant, 470 mg
Steak, 3 oz., 55 mg	**Corned beef**, 3 oz., 802 mg	**Jumbo burger**, fast food, 990 mg	**Meat loaf**, frozen dinner, 1,304 mg
Tomato, 14 mg	**Tomato juice**, 1 c., 878 mg	**Tomato soup**, 1 c., 932 mg	**Tomato sauce**, 1 c., 1, 498 mg
Tuna, fresh, 3 oz., 50 mg	**Tuna**, canned, 3 oz., 384 mg	**Tuna pot pie**, 1 frozen, 715 mg	**Fish sandwich**, 1, fast food, 882 mg
Peanuts, unsalted, 1 c., 8 mg	**Peanut butter**, 1 tbsp., 81 mg	**Peanut brittle**, 1 oz., 145 mg	**Dry roasted peanuts**, salted, 1 c., 986 mg

Sodium Labeling

Nutrition and ingredient labels on foods can show you the major sources of sodium in your diet and help you get an idea of your sodium intake.

Nutrition labels list the Daily Value (DV) for specific ingredients, including sodium. The DV for sodium is 2,400 mg. The sodium content of the food is listed in mg and as a percent of the daily value. The amount of sodium listed per serving includes sodium naturally present in the food as well as sodium added during processing.

Ingredients for all foods must be listed on the label, including standardized foods. Ingredients are listed in descending order by weight. Salt is the major, but not the only, source of sodium in food products. Any ingredient that has sodium, salt or soda as part of its name (monosodium glutamate, baking soda, seasoned salt) contains sodium. Soy sauce and other condiments used as ingredients also contribute sodium.

> Example -- INGREDIENTS: Potatoes, vegetable oil, whey, **salt**, dried milk solids, sour cream, **onion salt**, **monosodium glutamate**, dried parsley, lactic acid, **sodium citrate**, artificial flavors.

This food contains four sodium-containing ingredients (represented in bold above). Salt is the fourth ingredient by weight. Therefore, this product is probably high in sodium.

Specific health claims can be made about sodium for food products that meet certain requirements. For example, "A diet low in sodium may reduce the risk of high blood pressure, a disease associated with many factors." In order to make a health claim about sodium and hypertension (high blood pressure), the food must be low or very low in sodium. The following terms describe products that help reduce sodium intake:

- Sodium free: Less than 5 mg per serving.

- Very low sodium: 35 mg or less per serving and, if the serving is 30 g or less or 2 tablespoons or less, per 50 g of the food.

- Low sodium: 140 mg or less per serving and, if the serving is 30 g or less or 2 tablespoons or less, per 50 g of the food.

- Reduced or Less sodium: At least 25 percent less per serving than the reference food.

Steps to Reduce Sodium

One of the Dietary Guidelines for Americans is to avoid too much sodium. Use the following suggestions as starting points to reduce sodium in your diet.

- Learn to enjoy food's natural taste.

- Use natural unprocessed foods. The more processed the food is, the more sodium it may contain. Buy fresh or frozen vegetables, the canned ones have salt added.

- Use olive oil instead of butter or margarine in cooking.

- Check food labels for the words salt or sodium. Salt often is used as a preservative or flavoring agent. (See Table 2.)

- Season foods with herbs and spices rather than salt. (See Table 3.)

- **Do not use salt substitutes, especially those that contain potassium,**

- Check with your doctor or pharmacist for the sodium content of medications, especially antacids; cough medicines, laxatives and pain relievers.

- Try products such as low or reduced sodium to curb sodium intake

- Plan meals that contain less sodium. Try new recipes that use less salt and sodium-containing ingredients. Adjust your own recipes by reducing such ingredients a little at a time. Don't be fooled by recipes that have little or no salt added but call for ingredients like soups, bouillon cubes or condiments that do.

- Make your own condiments, dressings and sauces and keep sodium-containing ingredients at a minimum.

- Cut back on salt used in cooking pasta, rice, noodles, vegetables and hot cereals.

- Taste your food before you salt it. If, after tasting your food, you must salt it, try one shake instead of two.

- If using canned food, rinse in water to remove some of the salt before preparing or serving.

Table 2: Some high-sodium condiments

Onion salt	Baking soda	Mustard
Celery salt	Monosodium glutamate (MSG)	Worcestershire sauce
Garlic salt		Salad dressings
Seasoned salt	Soy sauce	Pickles
Meat tenderizer	Steak sauce	Chili sauce
Bouillon	Barbeque sauce	Relish
Baking powder	Catsup	

Table 3: Seasoning without your salt shaker use herbs and spice

For Appetizers

Hors d'oeuvres	Chervil, oregano, paprika, parsley
Cheese dips and spreads	Basil, chervil, dill weed, marjoram, oregano, sage, parsley, summer savory, tarragon
Deviled or stuffed eggs	Curry powder, dill weed, summer savory, tarragon
Dips	Curry powder, oregano, chervil, parsley
Mushrooms	Oregano, marjoram
Seafood cocktails and spreads	Basil, dill weed, thyme, bay leaves, tarragon

For Vegetables

Asparagus	Lemon peel, thyme
Broccoli	Lemon juice, onion
Brussels sprouts	Lemon juice, mustard
Cabbage	Dill weed, caraway seeds, oregano, lemon juice, vinegar, onion, mustard, marjoram

Carrots	Marjoram, ginger, mint, mace, parsley, nutmeg, sage, unsalted butter, lemon peel, orange peel, thyme, cinnamon
Cauliflower	Rosemary, nutmeg, tarragon, mace
Celery	Dill weed, tarragon
Cucumbers	Rosemary, onion
Green beans	Basil, dill weed, thyme, curry powder, lemon juice, vinegar
Peas	Mint, onion, parsley, basil, chervil, marjoram, sage, rosemary
Potatoes	Bay leaves, chervil, dill weed, mint, parsley, rosemary, paprika, tarragon, mace, nutmeg, unsalted butter, chives
Spinach	Chervil, marjoram, mint, rosemary, mace, nutmeg, lemon, tarragon
Squash	Basil, saffron, ginger, mace, nutmeg, orange peel
Tomatoes	Basil, bay leaves, chervil, tarragon, curry powder, oregano, parsley, sage, cloves
Zucchini	Marjoram, mint, saffron, thyme

For Entrees	
Eggs and cheese	Curry powder, marjoram, mace, parsley flakes, turmeric, basil, oregano, rosemary, garlic, mustard, mace, ginger, curry powder, allspice, lemon juice, pepper
Fish and shell-fish	Basil, bay leaves, chervil, marjoram, oregano, parsley, rosemary, sage, tarragon, thyme, lemon peel, celery seed, cumin, saffron, savory, dry mustard
Poultry	Basil, saffron, bay leaves, sage, dill weed, savory, marjoram, tarragon, oregano, thyme, rosemary, paprika, curry powder, orange peel, cranberries, mushrooms

For Fruits and Desserts	
Apples	Allspice, cardamom, ginger, cinnamon, cloves, nutmeg
Bananas	Allspice, ginger, cinnamon, nutmeg
Oranges	Allspice, cinnamon, anise, nutmeg, cloves, ginger, mace, rosemary
Pears	Allspice, cinnamon, nutmeg, anise, mint
Fruit compotes	Basil, rosemary, saffron, thyme
Puddings	Arrowroot, cinnamon, cloves, lemon peel, vanilla bean, ginger, mace, nutmeg, orange peel

DO NOT USE SALT SUBSTITUE SUCH AS LITE SALT, NO SALT. THE SALT SUBSTITUES CONTAIN POTASSIUM AND SHOULD BE AVOIDED. SOME LOWER SALT BOUILLON CUBES AND POWDERS ALSO USE POTASSIUM CHLORIDE AS A SALT SUBSTITUTE, READ THE LABELS.

Becoming an expert
label reader

The label below tells you that 1 bar contains 83 mg of sodium, therefore if you ate 4 bars (the entire package) you would consume 332 mg of sodium.

Nutrition Facts

Serving Size 1 Bar (85g)
Servings Per Container 4

Amount Per Serving

Calories 170   Calories from Fat 50

	% Daily Value *
Total Fat 6g	**9%**
Saturated Fat 4g	**19%**
Trans Fat 0g	
Polyunsaturated Fat 0.5g	
Monounsaturated Fat 1g	
Cholesterol 13mg	**4%**
Sodium 83mg	**3%**
Total Carbohydrate 33g	**11%**
Dietary Fiber 4g	**16%**
Sugar 25g	
Protein 3g	

Vitamin A 110%	•	Vitamin C 2%
Calcium 10%	•	Iron 3%

*Percent Daily Values are based on a 2,000 calorie diet. Your daily values may be higher or lower depending on your calorie needs.

	Calories	2,000	2,500
Total Fat	Less than	65g	80g
Sat Fat	Less than	20g	25g
Cholesterol	Less than	300mg	300mg
Sodium	Less than	2,400mg	2,400mg
Total Carbohydrate		300g	375g
Dietary Fiber		25g	30g

Calories per gram:
Fat 9   •   Carbohydrate 4   •   Protein 4

Is there a difference between
regular table salt, sea salt or kosher salt?

From a cooking perspective the main difference is texture. Table salt is very fine which makes it easy to dissolve. Sea salt and kosher salt are coarser and add a bit of crunch when seasoning last minute.

Chemically there isn't much difference unless you're buying iodized table salt (which of course has iodine added later).

Table salt is mined from underground salt deposits, and includes a small portion of calcium silicate, an anti-caking agent added to prevent clumping. It possesses very fine crystals and a sharp taste.

Sea salt is harvested from evaporated seawater and receives little or no processing; leaving intact the minerals from the water it came from.

Kosher salt takes its name from its use in the koshering process. It contains no preservatives and can be derived from either seawater or underground sources.

Many people believe that sea salt and kosher salt is healthier because of the way they are mined, they retain most of their minerals and some of the natural moisture that help the body.

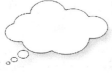 These different salts may have fewer added chemicals but as far as sodium and the potential to raise your blood pressure they are the same. All forms of salts need to be limited.

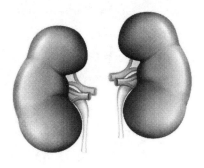

CHAPTER 5

STEP 2 DIABETES: CONTROL IT

If You Have It Control It

The two most common types of Diabetes are Type 1 also known as insulin dependent. All people with type 1 diabetes need to take insulin because their bodies don't make it any longer. Type two diabetes is initially controlled by diet, weight loss and exercise, medications, may be added to the regimen at a later time.

People who have been diagnosed with Diabetes may progress to Diabetic Nephropathy.

Diabetes is a serious disease and should be taken very seriously. I often see patients who tell me they "Have a touch of sugar". This touch of sugar can wreck havoc on their body and should be taken very seriously. The guidelines for blood sugar control are:

	GOAL	TAKE ACTION
Pre Meal or Fasting	< 100	< 70 Or > 130
2 Hours Post Prandial	< 140	> 180
Bedtime	70-130	< 110 > 160
A1c	6.5	> 7

These are firm guidelines and should be achieved with diet and medication if necessary. I see patients who will do anything to stay off insulin. One gentleman even cut out all grains, limited vegetables and fruits, all sources of carbohydrates that would increase his blood sugar level. If you cut all that out you only have fat and protein left and that is certainly not good for your kidneys and general health. If oral medication and a well balanced diet are not keeping your sugar in the recommended guidelines, insulin has to be considered.

High blood sugar wrecks havoc on you body and if insulin needs to be considered then please consider it. The consequences of untreated high blood sugar will be much worse that the tiny insulin needle.

One patient had poorly managed diabetes but refused to take insulin. He followed my diet and continued with oral meds as ordered by his physician. I saw him when his GFR was 48 and his HgA1c was 9. I saw him a year later and his GFR decreased to 37 and his HgA1c was 9.2. At this time he was alarmed and agreed to take insulin, follow my diet with much more diligence. I saw him 4 months later with no increase in GFR and an HgA1c of 7. One year later his GFR improved to 42 his HgA1c is 6.2 he felt great and his Ophthalmologist said that his eyes look much freer of Diabetic Retinopathy. He and his wife thanked me for bullying them into accepting insulin as a better way of managing his Diabetes.

Diabetic nephropathy

Diabetic nephropathy is kidney disease or damage that results as a complication of diabetes.

Causes

The exact cause of diabetic nephropathy is unknown, but it is believed that uncontrolled high blood sugar leads to the development of kidney damage. In some cases, your genes or family history may also play a role. Not all persons with diabetes develop this condition.

Each kidney is made of hundreds of thousands of filtering units called nephrons. Each nephron has a cluster of tiny blood vessels called a glomerulus. Together these structures help remove waste from the body. Too much blood sugar can damage these structures, causing them to thicken and become scarred. Slowly, over time, more and more blood vessels are destroyed. The kidney structures begin to leak and protein (albumin) begins to pass into the urine.

Persons with diabetes who have the following risk factors are more likely to develop this condition:

- African American, Hispanic, or American Indian origin

- Family history of kidney disease or high blood pressure

- Poor control of blood pressure

- Poor control of blood sugars

- Type 1 diabetes before age 20

- Smoking

Diabetic nephropathy generally goes along with other diabetes complications including high blood pressure, retinopathy, and blood vessel changes.

Symptoms: Early stage diabetic nephropathy has no symptoms. Over time, the kidney's ability to function may decline. Symptoms develop late in the disease and may include:

- Fatigue

- Foamy appearance or excessive frothing of the urine

- Frequent hiccups

- Generalized ill feeling

- Generalized itching

- headache

- nausea and vomiting

- poor appetite

- swelling of the feet and ankles

- Swelling, usually around the eyes in the mornings; general body swelling may occur with late-stage disease

- Unintentional weight gain (from fluid buildup)

Your doctor may think you have diabetic nephropathy if you have diabetes and a routine urinalysis shows too much protein in your urine. This test may also show glucose in the urine, especially if your blood sugar is poorly controlled.

The main sign of diabetic nephropathy is persistent protein in the urine. (Protein may appear in the urine for 5 to 10 years before other symptoms develop.) If your doctor thinks you might have this condition, a micro albuminuria test will be done. A positive test often means you have at least some damage to the kidney from diabetes. Damage at this stage may be reversible.

High blood pressure often goes along with diabetic nephropathy. You may have high blood pressure that develops rapidly or is difficult to control.

Laboratory tests that may be done include:

- BUN

- Serum Creatinine

The levels of these tests will increase, as kidney damage gets worse. Other laboratory tests that may be done include:

- 24-hour urine protein

- Blood levels of phosphorus, calcium, bicarbonate, and potassium

- Hemoglobin

- Hematocrit

- Red blood cell (RBC) count

A kidney biopsy confirms the diagnosis. However, your doctor can diagnose the condition without a biopsy if you meet the following three conditions:

1. Persistent protein in the urine

2. Diabetic retinopathy

3. No other kidney or renal tract disease

A biopsy may be done, however, if there is any doubt in the diagnosis.

Treatment

The goals of treatment are to keep the kidney disease from getting worse and prevent complications. This involves keeping your blood pressure under control (under 130/80). Controlling high blood pressure is the most effective way of slowing kidney damage from diabetic nephropathy.

Your doctor may prescribe the following medicines to lower your blood pressure:

- Angiotensin-converting enzyme (ACE) inhibitors

- Angiotensin receptor blockers (ARBs)

These drugs help reduce the amount of protein in the urine. Many studies have suggested that a combination of these two types of drugs may be best.

It is also very important to control lipid levels, maintain a healthy weight, and engage in regular physical activity.

You should closely monitor your blood sugar levels. Doing so may help slow down kidney damage, especially in the very early stages of the disease. Your can change your diet to help control your blood sugar. Your doctor may also prescribe medications to help control your blood sugar.

Your dosage of medicine may need to be adjusted from time to time. As kidney failure declines, your body may remove less insulin; so smaller doses may be needed to control glucose levels.

Urinary tract and other infections are common and can be treated with antibiotics.

DIABETES MEDICATIONS:
Take Control of your health

Medications may be taken individually or in combination pills.

Insulin, a hormone that is the natural substance your body uses to control blood glucose. If you have type 1 diabetes, your body can no longer make its own which is why you will have to inject your own insulin. Type two diabetics can manage the disease with diet, exercise and oral medications. Many will require insulin at some point.

Insulin comes in two basic types: shorter acting often called a bolus or mealtime insulin and long acting, basal insulin.

Shorter acting insulins: aspart (Novo Log), glulisine (Apidra), lispro (Humalog), and human regular insulin (Humulin R, Novolin R, Relion/Novolin R) are usually taken at mealtime and provide a quick burst of insulin to manage the glucose that surges into the blood stream after eating. Longer acting insulins NPH (Humulin N, Novolin N, Relion/Novolin N), glargine (Lantus) determir (Levemir) provide a lower background level of insulin to control blood glucose between meals and overnight. They are usually taken once or twice per day. Everyone with type 1 and many people with type 2 use both shorter and longer acting insulins, taken separately or in the same injections as a mixture.

ALPAH-GLUCOSIDASE INHIBITORS: Slow the breakdown of starches in the intestine, slowing down the excessive rise in blood glucose that happens after eating. Take with the first bite of your meal.

Possible side effects: Gas, diarrhea

Medications: acarbose known as Precose and miglitol known as Glyset

EXENATIDE: *Byetta, stimulates your own body to produce insulin. This is an injectible medication which needs to be taken an hour before the morning and evening meal. Possible side effects: short term nausea, weight loss.

* should not be taken by people with decreased kidney function (GFR < 30)

MEGLITINIDES: Increase insulin production by the pancreas. Taken before all three meals.

Possible side effects: hypoglycemia.

Available forms: nateglinide (Starlix) and repaglinide (Prandin)

*METFORMIN: decreases the liver's glucose output and increases the uptake of glucose by muscles. Taken one to three times per day or available in extended release formula (XR), which is taken once per day.

Possible side effects: nauseas, upset stomach, diarrhea (lessened when taken with food or the XR formula).

*Medications available: metformin (Fortamet, Glucophage, Glucophage XR, Gumetza, Riomet)

* should not be taken by people with decreased kidney function

PRAMLINTIDE ACETATE: (Synlin) an injected medication that can reduce a person's insulin requirement. Symlin is an analogue of a naturally occurring hormone that is released by the pancreas and helps with blood glucose control. Approved for both type 1 and 2 diabetes.

Possible side effects: nausea usually gets better with time.

SITAGLIPTIN: (Januvia) stimulates insulin production by the pancreas. Taken once a day with or without food.

SULFONYUREAS: stimulate insulin production by the pancreas. Taken once or twice before meals.

Possible side effects: hypoglycemia may react with alcohol.

Medications available: glimepiride (**Amaryl), glipizide ***Glucotrol, ***Glucotrol XL) glyburide (*Diabeta, Glynase Pres Tab, *Micronase) chlororomie (*Diabinase)
* should not be taken by people with decreased kidney function (GFR<50)
** GFR < 22 starting dose smaller
**** should not be taken by people with decreased kidney function (GFR <10)

THIAZOLIDINEDIONES: also known as TZD's they enhance the action of the body's own insulin in muscle and fat, plus reduce glucose production by the liver. Taken with or without food.

Possible side effects: water retention, weight gain, congestive heart failure.

Medications available: pioglitazone (Actos) and rosiglitazone (Avandia).

Steps to manage
your medications effectively

1. Know exactly what medication you are on.

2. Make a schedule, if you are taking a lot of medications you may need to figure out how they all fit together.

3. Avoid bad interactions. Some medications should not be taken together. Some should not be taken with fruit juices (grapefruit juice in particular). Your pharmacist may be very helpful with minimizing interactions.

4. Never skip a dose, never double up to catch up

Changing the Diet

The principles of a diabetic diet begin with

1. Strive to attain a more desirable body weight. Even a modest weight loss can help stabilize blood glucose levels.

2. Try for consistent meal times and consistent balance of carbohydrates, protein and fats. The plate method, which is described below, can help with managing those proportions.

3. Increase fiber in the diet.

4. Plan for at least 30 minutes of exercise daily.

5. Check blood glucose levels daily, I especially recommend two hours after meals to help you determine if that meal promoted the desired 2 hour post meal goal 140-180

6. Work with your physician to manage your medications to achieve target blood glucose levels and HgA1c

7. Select olive oil as the preferred oil

Read labels:

Read the labels look make sure that added sugars are not listed as one of the first few ingredients. Other names for added sugars include: corn syrup, high-fructose corn syrup, fruit juice concentrate, maltose, dextrose, sucrose, honey, and maple syrup.

Plain Yogurt

Nutrition Facts

Serving Size: 1 cup (8 fl oz) (245g)

Amount Per Serving

Calories 149	Calories from Fat 72

% Daily Value*

Total Fat 7.96 g	12%
Saturated Fat 5.14 g	26%
Trans Fat	
Cholesterol 31.85 mg	11%
Sodium 112.7 mg	5%
Potassium 379.75 mg	11%
Total Carbohydrate 11.42 g	4%
Dietary Fiber 0 g	0%
Sugars 11.42 g	
Sugar Alcohols	
Protein 8.5 g	
Vitamin A 242.55 IU	5%
Vitamin C 1.23 mg	2%
Calcium 296.45 mg	30%
Iron 0.12 mg	1%

Fruit Yogurt

Nutrition Facts

Serving Size: 1 cup (8 fl oz) (245g)

Amount Per Serving

Calories 243	Calories from Fat 25

% Daily Value*

Total Fat 2.82 g	4%
Saturated Fat 1.82 g	9%
Trans Fat	
Cholesterol 12.25 mg	4%
Sodium 129.85 mg	5%
Potassium 433.65 mg	12%
Total Carbohydrate 45.67 g	15%
Dietary Fiber 0 g	0%
Sugars 45.67 g	
Sugar Alcohols	
Protein 9.75 g	
Vitamin A 98 IU	2%
Vitamin C 1.47 mg	2%
Calcium 338.1 mg	34%
Iron 0.15 mg	1%

Now look below at the ingredient lists for the two yogurts. Ingredients are listed in descending order of weight (from most to least). Note that no added sugars or sweeteners are in the list of ingredients for the plain yogurt, yet 10g of sugars were listed on the Nutrition Facts label. This is because there are no added sugars in plain yogurt, only naturally occurring sugars (lactose in the milk).

Plain Yogurt - contains no added sugars

INGREDIENTS: CULTURED PASTEURIZED GRADE A NONFAT MILK, WHEY PROTEIN CONCENTRATE, PECTIN, CARRAGEENAN.

Fruit Yogurt - contains added sugars

INGREDIENTS: CULTURED GRADE A REDUCED FAT MILK, APPLES, HIGH FRUCTOSE CORN SYRUP, CINNAMON, NUTMEG, NATURAL FLAVORS, AND PECTIN. CONTAINS ACTIVE YOGURT AND L. ACIDOPHILUS CULTURES.

Create Your Plate

Often, when people are diagnosed with diabetes, they don't know where to begin. One way is to change the amount of food you are already eating. Focus on filling your plate with non-starchy vegetables and having smaller portions of starchy foods and animal protein. Creating your plate is an easy way to get started with managing blood glucose levels.

You don't need any special tools or have to do any counting. It's simple and effective — draw an imaginary line on your plate, select your foods, and enjoy your meal! The easiest way to get started with managing your diabetes is to create your plate.

It's simple and effective for both managing diabetes and losing weight. Creating your plate lets you still choose the foods you want, but changes the portion sizes so you are getting larger portions of non-starchy vegetables and a smaller portion of starchy foods. When you are ready, you can try new foods within each food category.

Try these 6 simple steps to get started:

1. Using your dinner plate put a line down the middle of the plate.

2. Then on one side, cut it again so you will have 3 sections on your plate.

3. Fill the largest section with non starchy vegetables such as:

   Asparagus, bamboo shoots, beets, bok choy broccoli cabbage, carrots, cauli-flower, celery, cucumber eggplant, green beans iceberg lettuce, onion, okra, mushrooms

4. Now in one of the small sections, put starchy foods such as:
   - whole grain breads, such as whole wheat or rye
   - whole grain, high-fiber cereal
   - cooked cereal such as oatmeal, grits, hominy, or cream of wheat
   - rice, *pasta, dal, tortillas
   - cooked beans and peas, such as pinto beans or black- eyed peas
   - rice, green peas, corn, lima beans, winter squash, pasta
   - low-fat crackers and snack chips, pretzels, and fat-free popcorn
     * lower glycemic pasta: Dreamfields brand. In my area regular grocery stores carry it in the pasta section.

5. And then on the other small section, put your protein such as:

- chicken or turkey without the skin

- fish such as tuna, salmon, cod, or catfish

- other seafood such as shrimp, clams, oysters, crab, o r mussels

- tofu, eggs, low-fat cheese

6. Add a 4 oz. glass off non-fat milk. If you don't drink milk, you can add another small serving of carb such as a 6 oz. container of light yogurt or a small roll.

7. And a piece of fruit or a 1/2 cup fruit salad and you have your meal planned. Examples are fresh, frozen, or canned in juice.

Breakfast

Your plate will look different at breakfast but the idea is the same. If you use a plate or bowl for breakfast, keep your portions small. Use half your plate for starchy foods. You can ad fruit in the small part and a meat or meat substitute in the other.

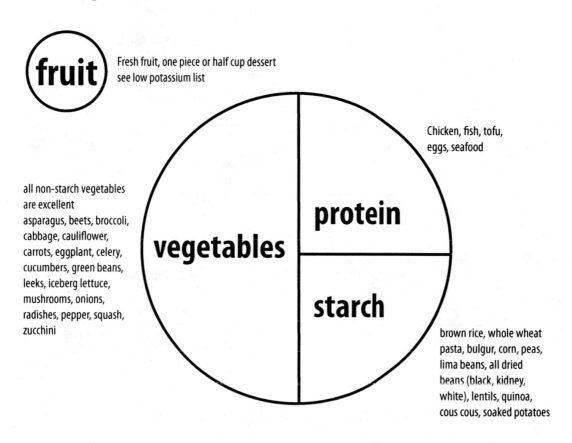

Fresh fruit, one piece or half cup dessert see low potassium list

Chicken, fish, tofu, eggs, seafood

all non-starch vegetables are excellent asparagus, beets, broccoli, cabbage, cauliflower, carrots, eggplant, celery, cucumbers, green beans, leeks, iceberg lettuce, mushrooms, onions, radishes, pepper, squash, zucchini

brown rice, whole wheat pasta, bulgur, corn, peas, lima beans, all dried beans (black, kidney, white), lentils, quinoa, cous cous, soaked potatoes

The vegetables are from the low and moderate potassium lists, protein from the recommended list.

Meal Planning with the Plate Method

Lunch/Dinner

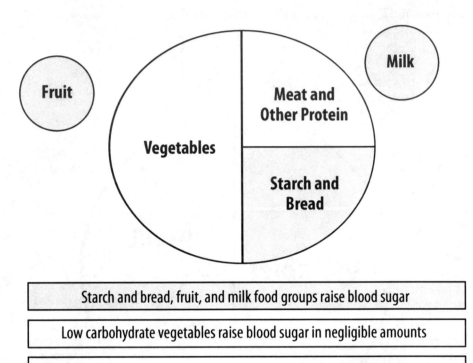

Starch and bread, fruit, and milk food groups raise blood sugar
Low carbohydrate vegetables raise blood sugar in negligible amounts
Meat and protein foods raise blood sugar very little with moderate portions

What raises your blood glucose level? Infection, stress, eating sweets

What are affects your daily blood glucose level? Diet, exercise and high fiber diet.

Select from the foods in the chart on the next page to add fiber to your diet

FOOD	AMOUNT	TOTAL FIBER (Grams)
Avocado*	1 medium	11.84
Black beans, cooked*	1 cup	14.92
Bran cereal	1 cup	19.94
Broccoli, cooked	1 cup	4.5
Green peas, cooked*	1 cup	8.84
Kale, cooked	1 cup	7.20
Kidney beans, cooked*	1 cup	13.33
Lentils, cooked*	1 cup	15.64
Lima beans, cooked*	1 cup	13.16
Navy beans, cooked*	1 cup	11.65
Oats, dry	1 cup	12.00
Pinto beans, cooked*	1 cup	14.71
Split peas, cooked*	1 cup	16.27
Raspberries	1 cup	8.34
Rice, brown, uncooked	1 cup	7.98
Soybeans, cooked	1 cup	7.62
Almonds*	1 oz.	4.22
Apples, w/skin	1 medium	5.00
Banana*	1 medium	3.92
Blueberries	1 cup	4.18

FOOD	AMOUNT	TOTAL FIBER (Grams)
Cabbage, cooked	1 cup	4.20
Cauliflower, cooked	1 cup	3.43
Corn, sweet	1 cup	4.66
Flax seeds	3 tsp	6.97
Garbanzo beans, cooked*	1 cup	5.80
Grapefruit*	1/2 medium	6.12
Green beans, cooked	1 cup	3.95
Olives	1 cup	4.30
Oranges, navel*	1 medium	3.40
Papaya*	1 each	5.47
Pasta, whole wheat	1 cup	6.34
Peach, dried*	3 pcs.	3.18
Pear	1 medium	5.08
Pistachio nuts*	1 oz.	3.10
Potato, baked w/ skin*	1 medium	4.80
Prunes*	1/4 cup	3.02
Pumpkin seeds*	1/4 cup	4.12
Sesame seeds	1/4 cup	4.24
Spinach, cooked*	1 cup	4.32
Strawberries	1 cup	3.98

*high potassium

This meal and blood glucose grid is for you to keep each day. Take a look and identify when your blood glucose is too high or too low. Does your diet need tweaking? Is your medication working for you?

Blood Glucose log TARGET BLOOD GLUCOSE

	GOAL	TAKE ACTION
PRE MEAL OR FASTING	< 100	< 70 OR > 130
2 HOURS POST PRANDIAL	< 140	> 180
BED TIME	70-130	< 110 > 160
A1c	6.5	> 7

FASTING B.G	BREAKFAST	INSULIN DOSE	2 HR B.G	LUNCH	INSULIN DOSE	2 HR B.G	DINNER	INSULIN DOSE	2 HR B.G	NITE B.G

KNOW YOUR A1C

In addition to testing your blood sugar regularly, you should know your A1C.

What is a Hemoglobin A1C Test? (HGB A1C)?

This is a very useful blood test, done by the laboratory to estimate blood sugar levels for the past 3 months. Hemoglobin is a red blood cell that has a lifespan of approximately 90 days. The glucose in your blood attaches itself to a red blood cell (Hgb). The amount that attaches to the Hgb depends on how high the blood glucose is. For example, if glucose is high, more of it attaches to the red blood cell; if glucose is low, very little attaches. The glucose stays attached until the hemoglobin molecule is broken down naturally by the body, approximately 90 days. The amount of hemoglobin with glucose attached is measured. This indicates how high the blood glucose has been, over the past 3 months. For instance, if your glucose was high one month ago, then more glucose would have attached to the hemoglobin molecule at that time, and this could still be measured now. Measuring the HgbA1c is a convenient way for your doctor to get more information about your glucose control, and to track your progress. It becomes easy to whether overall glucose control is actually improving, or worsening. Excellent levels, for someone with diabetes, would be 7.0% (.070) or less of total hemoglobin having glucose attached. When your HgbA1c is good, you can be sure that your glucose levels have been good for a long time.

Target HgA1C

You and your doctor will decide what your target A1C should be. For most people with diabetes, the American Diabetes Association recommends an A1C of less than 7%. Another group of experts, the American Association of Clinical Endocrinologists, recommends an even lower A1C of 6.5% or less.

How much can you lower your risk of complications?

- In type 2 diabetes, every 1% drop in A1c lowers the risk of complications by 37%!

- In type 1 diabetes, lowering the A1c from 9% to 7% reduced complications by 34-76%!

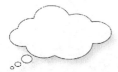 By improving your glycemic control you will be improving the outcome of your kidney health.

Some research on beneficial supplementation with Diabetes.

CHROMIUM

The benefit of chromium supplements for diabetes has been studied and debated for a few years. Clinical studies have reported that chromium supplements may reduce blood sugar levels as well as the amount of insulin needed. Chromium was found to reduce insulin resistance, especially in people who smoke. Chromium is an antioxidant that helps protect the body against free radical damage also known as oxidation.

The recommended level for chromium is 30 mcg per day.

MAGNESIUM

Type 2 diabetes is associated with low levels of magnesium in the blood. Magnesium has been found to improve insulin sensitivity. Magnesium deficiency in diabetic patients may decrease their immunity making them more susceptible to infections and illness. Green vegetables, legumes, peas, nuts and whole grains are good sources

The recommended intake of Magnesium is 400 mg per day.

L CARNITINE

When high blood sugar levels damage nerves in the body, especially the arms, legs and feet the condition is called diabetic neuropathy. Some small preliminary studies suggest that L Carnitine may help reduce the pain and increase normal feelings in affected nerves.

The recommended dose of 3 grams daily for 1 year.

VITAMINS

Look for multivitamins that give only 100% RDA's with additional Magnesium Zinc and Chromium.

Know your sugars

The following sweeteners are forms of "sugar" they have different sources and processing methods but what they do have in common is that they all cause your blood glucose to rise and should be thought of as sugar.

White Sugars

"Regular" or white table sugar, from coarse to powdered granulations there are many different types of refined, granulated sugar derived from sugar cane or sugar beets. Cane and beet sugars are mainly made of sucrose and come in varying crystal sizes that provide unique functional characteristics appropriate for a specific food's special need.

Refined white sugar is 50% glucose and 50% fructose, and is highly processed using multiple fossil fuel and chemical-intensive processes. It provides empty calories and zero nutritional value. Additionally, the fact that **over 65% of commercial sugar is made from genetically engineered (GMO) sugar beets** makes white sugar something **to be avoided at all costs.**

"Fruit Sugar" or Crystalline Fructose Crystalline fructose is slightly finer than "regular" sugar and is used in dry mixes such as flavored gelatin and pudding desserts, and powdered drinks. Crystalline fructose has a more uniform small crystal size than "regular" sugar which prevents separation or settling of larger crystals to the bottom of the box—an important quality in dry mixes. Since it is made totally from fructose, it is definitely harmful to your health.

Brown Sugars

Brown sugars range in the amount of processing they receive, but they are brown because, unlike white sugar, they have not had all of the molasses chemically and physically removed. The least processed of the brown sugars—Rapadura or panela—often still has the minerals and enzymes intact.

Brown palm sugars differ in texture and taste from brown cane sugars, but are often minimally processed as to still contain trace minerals too. Brown sugars can be used in cup-for-cup substitution with white refined sugars.

Brown Sugar (common light and dark) Common brown sugar is really highly processed and refined white sugar that has had the surface molasses syrup added back in, which imparts its characteristic flavor.

Turbinado is raw sugar that has been partially processed, where only the surface molasses has been washed off. It has a blond color and mild brown sugar flavor, and is often used in tea and other beverages. Sugar in the Raw™ is the most commonly known brand of raw, turbinado sugar.

Liquid Sugars

Corn syrup: converted cornstarch into an alternative sweetener called *high fructose corn syrup*. High fructose corn syrup contains 55% fructose and 45% glucose, which make it virtually as sweet as sucrose or natural honey. When imported sugar became prohibitively expensive, many processed food and beverage manufacturers began using high fructose corn syrup exclusively.

Today, high fructose corn syrup has replaced pure sugar as the main sweetener in most carbonated beverages, including Coca Cola and Pepsi products. High fructose corn syrup is also hiding in products like salad dressing, spaghetti sauce, and whole wheat bread, and it is often one of the first ingredients in cake mixes, cookies, sauces, breakfast cereals and commercial baked goods.

High fructose corn syrup is made through a highly industrialized, chemical fermentation and distillation process that uses tremendous amounts of energy to produce. Many health experts and environmentalists are concerned over the level of genetic modification, environmental pollution and toxic processing used to create high fructose corn syrup. High fructose corn syrup is extremely glycemic.

Agave Syrup

Agave syrup is very high in fructose. Depending on the brand, agave can contain as much as 92% fructose. Nowhere in nature does this ratio of fructose to glucose occur naturally. The amount of fructose in agave is much, much higher than the 55% fructose in high-fructose corn syrup or the 50% fructose in refined table sugar, making agave "nectar" worse for you than either table sugar or corn syrup.

The fact that agave syrup is high in low-glycemic fructose is often hailed as a benefit of using it. What many people don't realize is that concentrated fructose is probably worse for you than high amounts of glucose. In fact, agave syrup has been banned by the Glycemic Index Institute for the harm it caused to study participants.

Agave is not naturally sweet like sugar cane, honey or fruit. Whether heavily processed with heat and chemicals or minimally processed with enzymes, agave syrup requires an industrial process to extract its sweetness. As such, agave syrup is not a whole or traditional food. It is a factory-made, modern product, and like all processed foods, agave syrup is missing many of the enzymes and nutrients that the original plant had to begin with.

And like many processed foods, it contains very high amounts of fructose that the human body simply wasn't designed to handle.

Rice Syrup Rice syrup is a natural sweetener, which is made from, cooked brown rice which is specially fermented to turn the starches in the rice into sugars. Along with other alternatives to sugar, rice syrup can usually be found in natural foods stores and in some large markets. Since rice syrup will cause an elevation in blood sugar, it is not suitable for diabetics.

Apple Juice Concentrate 60% fructose, 27% glucose, 13% sucrose. It is made by cooking down apple juice until it is highly concentrated. The end result very sweet and causes a sharp rise in blood glucose level.

Honey

Honey is a mixture of sugars and other compounds, mainly fructose and glucose. Honey contains trace amounts of several vitamins and minerals and also contains tiny amounts of several compounds thought to function as antioxidants and anti-microbials. Despite being thought of as more natural, honey has an glycemic effect similar to white table sugar.

Sugar Alcohols

Xylitol, Erythritol, Mannitol, Sorbitol and Glycerine (Glycerol)

Sugar alcohols (which end in *-ol*) occur naturally in plants. Some of them are chemically or biologically extracted from plants (sorbitol from corn syrup and mannitol from seaweed), but they are mostly manufactured in a highly-intensive industrial process from sugars and starches.

Sugar alcohols are like sugar in some ways, but they are not completely absorbed by the body. Because of this, they affect blood sugar levels less, and they provide fewer calories per gram. Additionally, sugar alcohols don't promote tooth decay as sugars do, so are often used to sweeten "sugar-free" chewing gum.

Xylitol and erythritol can often be swapped one for one with sugar, but you will have to read the package and experiment with each type to see how it best substitutes for sugar in your recipes. Sugar alcohols do not brown or caramelize like sugars do.

Though sugar alcohols have fewer calories than sugar, most of them aren't as sweet, so more must be used to get the same sweetening effect. Still, there is a range of sweetness and impact on blood sugar among the sugar alcohols.

For example, *Maltitol* has 75% of the blood sugar impact of sugar, but only 75% of the sweetness, so they end up being equal in the end. *Xylitol* is just as sweet as cane sugar, but has a low glycemic index of 13, and also helps prevent tooth decay by inhibiting bacterial growth in the mouth. *Erythritol* is only 70% as sweet as cane sugar, but it has zero glycemic index, and is sometimes recommended for people fighting candida. *Food-grade glycerine*/glycerol is a liquid derived from vegetable oils, but it is only 60% as sweet as cane sugar, and can be hard to use.

Because they are not completely absorbed, sugar alcohols like sorbitol and xylitol can ferment in the intestines and cause bloating, gas, or diarrhea, and *they are not recommended for people with IBS or other digestive issues.*

Swerve® Swerve is the latest "natural sweetener" to hit the market. Swerve is made from a combination of erythritol, oligosaccharides and natural flavors that give it excellent baking and cooking functionality. Unlike other sugar alcohols, Swerve even has the ability to brown and caramelize!

Unfortunately, while preferable to artificial sweeteners like Equal, Sweet'N Low, and Splenda, Swerve is still a highly-refined sweetening agent made from a sugar alcohol. Even though it is generally recognized as safe (GRAS) by the U.S. Food and Drug Administration (FDA), erythritol has been known to cause stomach pains, headaches, and even diarrhea in some individuals.

However, erythritol is non-glycemic and non-carcinogenic. The company that produces Swerve claims it is non-allergenic and much less likely than other sugar alcohols to cause gastrointestinal distress. Even so, it is still a sugar alcohol, which means it is not completely absorbed by the body, and therefore has no nutritional benefits.

Sugar substitutes are available in a variety of forms. They are not to be thought of as a health food but have been seen as a positive addition to the diabetic diet. They help us manage the sweet tooth without affecting our blood sugar levels. In moderation they can be used safely.

Saccharin, first produced in 1970 it is the older of the artificial sweeteners. This sweetener used to have a warning label on it regarding tumor growth but that has been revoked since more than 30 human studies reported no saccharin-tumor grown connection. Some report a bitter after taste. You can bake with it.

Aspartame: Equal or NutraSweet. The American Diabetic Association maintains that this substance is safe. Not recommended for high temperature baking.

Sucralose: Splenda, on the market since 1998. Despite negative press there have been no serious adverse events reported. A large study at Duke University found reduced microbes in the feces in participants who used large quantities of Splenda. If that is something that might concern you then a daily probiotic may offset this. According to the FDA it is safe. Splenda can be used for baking.

Stevia: Sold as Truvia, Purevia, SweetLeaf. Some people report a licorice like after taste. Received FDA approval in 2008. Can be used for baking.

I encourage you to try the different sweeteners in your beverages and other places that you can't live without sugar. The goal is to reduce your intake of refined carbohydrates, reduce calories (if applicable) and these sugar substitutes can help you do both.

I have to tell you the story of a patient I saw, he came in eating chips and drinking a regular soda. When I recommended that he switches to a diet soda he said "that stuff in not good for you". I find it ironic that he would be telling me this while consuming lots of unpronounceable chemicals in the chips and causing a glucose surge to his blood stream from the soda. *I can't promise that in 50 years we will discover that these sweeteners are not the best but I can tell you that consuming excess sugar will be harmful today. Moderation is the key.*

The other words of wisdom I want to leave this chapter with are: Once you have adapted your diet to the plate method and you have kept your blood glucose log and found that you have high blood glucose levels after some meals. **The key is that the medication has to match your meals not your meals matching your medications.** If your diet is healthy, you are exercising regularly and your blood sugar goals are still not met. At this time an assessment of your medications may need to be useful.

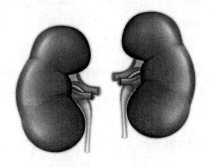

CHAPTER 6

STEP 3 MODIFY YOUR PROTEIN INTAKE

Protein- What Does It Do?

- Protein is necessary for the building and repair of body tissues.

- It produces enzymes, hormones, and other substances the body uses.

- It regulates body processes, such as water balancing, transporting nutrients, and making muscles contract.

- Protein keeps the body healthy by resisting diseases that are common to malnourished people.

- Prevents one from becoming easily fatigued by producing stamina and energy.

Protein comes mostly from meat but can also be found in eggs, milk, nuts, beans, and other foods. Healthy kidneys take wastes out of the blood but leave in the protein.

Impaired kidneys may fail to separate the protein from the wastes.

I calculate your protein needs based upon protein requirements of healthy individuals, I am not putting you on a low protein diet but a healthy level that we followed once upon a time before restaurant super-sizing and the birth of the American steak house.

The recommended levels of protein are based on IDEAL BODY WEIGHT. So first you have to determine your IBW using height weight charts or body mass index charts.

Height & Weight Table For Women

Height Feet Inches	Small Frame	Medium Frame	Large Frame
4' 10"	102-111	109-121	118-131
4' 11"	103-113	111-123	120-134
5' 0"	104-115	113-126	122-137
5' 1"	106-118	115-129	125-140
5' 2"	108-121	118-132	128-143
5' 3"	111-124	121-135	131-147
5' 4"	114-127	124-138	134-151
5' 5"	117-130	127-141	137-155
5' 6"	120-133	130-144	140-159
5' 7"	123-136	133-147	143-163
5' 8"	126-139	136-150	146-167
5' 9"	129-142	139-153	149-170
5' 10"	132-145	142-156	152-173
5' 11"	135-148	145-159	155-176
6' 0"	138-151	148-162	158-179

Weight in pounds according to frame (in indoor clothing weighing 3 lbs, with shoes with 1" heels)

Height & Weight Table For Men

Height Feet Inches	Small Frame	Medium Frame	Large Frame
5' 2"	128-134	131-141	138-150
5' 3"	130-136	133-143	140-153
5" 4"	132-138	135-145	142-156
5' 5"	134-140	137-148	144-160
5' 6"	136-142	139-151	146-164
5' 7"	138-145	142-154	149-168
5' 8"	140-148	145-157	152-172
5' 9"	142-151	148-160	155-176
5' 10"	144-154	151-163	158-180
5' 11"	146-157	154-166	161-184
6' 0"	149-160	157-170	164-188
6' 1"	152-164	160-174	168-192
6' 2"	155-168	164-178	172-197
6' 3"	158-172	167-182	176-202
6' 4"	162-176	171-187	181-207

Weight in pounds according to frame (in indoor clothing weighing 5 lbs.; shoes with 1" heels)

If you are close to your ideal body weight use your actual weight but if you are more than 10 lbs above Ideal Body Weight then find your ideal weight on the charts above and continue with the formula below.

How to Calculate Your Protein Needs:

Convert your weight to kilograms

1. Weight in pounds divided by 2.2 = weight in kilograms

2. Weight in kg x 0.8 = amount of protein you can eat per day

   Example: 154 lb male

   154 lbs divided by 2.2 = 70 kg
   70 kg x 0.8 = 56 gm protein/day.

This person should eat 56 grams of protein per day.

TO CALCULATE HOW MUCH PROTEIN YOU MAY EAT PER DAY: Lets say that you calculated your protein needs to be 65 grams per day how do you go about deciding what you can eat. To make matters just a bit more complicated 85-90% should come from animal based protein and the rest from vegetables and grains.

Step 1. 150 lb woman whose **ideal body weight** is 135 lbs.

Step 2. Convert to kilograms:

   135 lbs divided by 2.2 = 61.1 kilograms (kg)

Step 3 How much protein can I consume: 61.1 kg x 0.8 = 48.8 we can round to 49 grams protein per day

Step 4. How much protein from animal foods: 49 x 85% = 41.6 we can round to 42 grams of protein per day.

A deck of cards of animal protein is equivalent to 3 oz which provides 24 grams of protein. So to meet the goal of consuming 42 grams of protein per day I would suggest 2oz of animal protein at lunch (16 grams of protein) and 3 oz at dinner (24 grams protein)

See table in this chapter for protein content of common foods.

I will also tell you that to consume adequate calories and not find this diet overly monotonous I have people go over the protein level from grains and vegetables often I am strict with animal based protein but liberal with plant based protein

I further limit red meat from the diet as it has shown in studies to increase albuminuria (protein found in urine)

Table of protein content of foods

Foods	Protein Content
Ostrich	10 grams/ounce
Beef	7 grams/ounce
Poultry	7 grams/ounce
Fish	7 grams/ounce
Large Egg	7 grams/egg
Milk	8 grams/cup
Cheese (eg. Cheddar)	7 grams/ounce
Bread	4 grams/slice
Cereal	4 grams/1/2 cup
Vegetables	2 grams/ 1/2 cup
Soybeans (dry)	10 grams/ounce
Peanuts	7 grams/ounce
Lentils (dry)	6.5 grams/ounce
Red beans	6 grams/ounce
Baked potato	9 grams/8 ounces
Cashews	5 grams/ounce

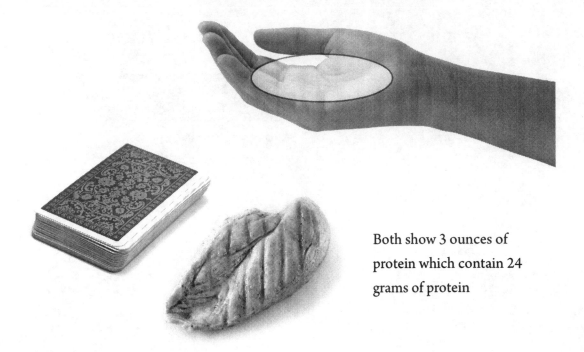

Both show 3 ounces of
protein which contain 24
grams of protein

Sample day to accommodate this protein level.

Breakfast

¾ cup of oatmeal with honey 1 cup raspberries

Snack

4 marshmallows

Lunch

Turkey sandwich: 2 slices of bread with 2 oz of turkey, lettuce,
tomato, mayo and mustard

1 c tossed salad with assorted vegetables Italian olive oil vinaigrette

1 c home made chicken soup

1   cup strawberries and cool whip

    Green tea

Dinner

3   oz. salmon

1   cup of green beans with olive oil garlic and Parmesan cheese

1   cup of rice with seasonings

    Tossed salad with olive oil and vinegar Rice krispies

4   oz red wine

This totals 35 grams of protein from animal based foods giving me 6 grams more for grains and vegetables. I know that I went over but a s I said the focus is mostly on animal based protein and less on protein from plant sources.

Sample Menus:

Breakfast	Breakfast	Breakfast	Breakfast
1 cup Rice Krispies cereal ½ c rice milk 1 cup blueberries coffee or tea	2 eggs whole wheat toast butter, jelly pineapple coffee or tea	8 oz cheerios almond milk cup strawberries coffee or tea	1 cup oatmeal with butter and brown sugar coffee and tea
Lunch	**Lunch**	**Lunch**	**Lunch**
2 oz Chicken Salad on bed of iceberg lettuce with carrots and cucumbers Balsamic and olive oil wheat roll, butter pineapple green tea	Home made additive free lower sodium chicken noodle soup With chunks of chicken Iceberg, cucumber, celery salad with Italian dressing Graham crackers 7 UP	Chef salad: iceberg lettuce, eggs, green beans, cheddar cheese, Balsamic vinaigrette Vanilla wafers Iced tea	Tuna sandwich on wheat bread Salad Animal crackers Water with lemon

Dinner	Dinner	Dinner	Dinner
2 cups pasta sautéed with green beans and broccoli using olive oil and garlic. Sprinkle with parmesan cheese	Scallops Snap Peas Rice Red wine	Home prepared stir Fried rice with egg and, green beans, carrots, corn and peas.	6 oz ground turkey meatloaf 1 cup mashed potatoes using soaked potatoes 1 cup asparagus white wine
Snack low salt popcorn	**Snack** Unsalted crackers with low sodium cheese	**Snack** sorbet	**Snack** popsicle

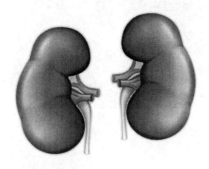

CHAPTER 7

STEP 4 MANAGE
YOUR POTASSIUM

Potassium is an element (and an electrolyte) that's essential for the body's growth and maintenance. It's necessary to keep a normal water balance between the cells and body fluids. Potassium also plays an essential role in the response of nerves to stimulation and in the contraction of muscles. Cellular enzymes need potassium to work properly.

Potassium is found naturally in many fruits and vegetables, such as oranges, potatoes, bananas, dried fruits, dried beans and peas, and nuts. Healthy kidneys measure potassium in the blood and remove excess amounts. Diseased kidneys may fail to remove excess potassium. With very poor kidney function, high potassium levels can affect the heart rhythm.

**If your potassium becomes too high, it can cause
an irregular heartbeat or a heart attack.**

What is a safe level of potassium in my blood?

If it is 3.5-5.0 . . . . You are in the **SAFE** zone

If it is 5.1-5.5 . . . . You are in the **CAUTION** zone

If it is higher than 6.0 . . . . You are in the **DANGER** zone

These are the guidelines recommended by the National Kidney Foundation. Some physicians have more stringent guidelines so ask your physician what his guidelines are.

List of Foods High in Potassium

Foods with Potassium	Serving Size	Potassium (mg)
Apricots, dried	10 halves	407
Avocados, raw	1 ounce	180
Bananas, raw	1 cup	594
Beets, cooked	1 cup	519
Brussel sprouts, cooked	1 cup	504
Cantaloupe	1 cup	494
Dates, dry	5 dates	271
Figs, dry	2 figs	271
Kiwi fruit, raw	1 medium	252

Foods with Potassium	Serving Size	Potassium (mg)
Lima beans	1 cup	955
Melons, honeydew	1 cup	461
Milk, fat free or skim	1 cup	407
Nectarines	1 nectarine	288
Orange juice	1 cup	496
Oranges	1 orange	237
Pears (fresh)	1 pear	208
Peanuts dry roasted, unsalted	1 ounce	187
Potatoes, baked, white, sweet, yams	1 potato	1081
Prune juice	1 cup	707
Prunes, dried	1 cup	828
Raisins	1 cup	1089
Spinach, cooked	1 cup	839
Tomato products, canned sauce	1 cup	909
Winter squash	1 cup	896

Fruit choices a serving is
1 piece of fruit or 1 cup

Daily selection (less than 100 mg per serving)	Twice per week (100-200 mg per serving)	Not recommended (200 mg or more per serving)
Apples and applesauce	Cantaloupe	Dried apricots
Blackberries	Cherries	Canned apricots
Blueberries	Clementine	Avocado
Pears	Craisins	Banana
Pineapple	Grapes	Dates
Raspberries	Mandarin orange	Figs
Strawberries	Papaya	Kiwi
Watermelon	Plum	Honey dew melon
	Tangerine	Prunes
	Canned peach	Raisins
		Rhubarb
		Orange
		Prune juice
		Orange juice
		Tropical juices
		Tomato juice

Vegetable choices: Low and moderate potassium
a serving is ½ c cooked or 1 cup raw.

Daily selection	Three times per week	Not recommended
Green beans	Asparagus	Arugula
Wax beans	Beets	Beet greens
Carrots	Boston lettuce ½ c	Brussel sprouts
Cucumber	Broccoli	Black eyed peas
Endive	Cabbage	Parsnip
Escarole	Cauliflower	Potato
Iceberg lettuce	Celery	Soy beans
Green peas	Eggplant	Spinach
2 slices tomato	Kale	Winter squash
	Lime beans	Tomato sauce
	Mushrooms	Yam
	Okra	
	Onions	
	Green peppers	
	Radish	
	Summer squash	
	Soaked potatoes	

Leaching potassium out of vegetables

The process of leaching will help pull potassium out of some high-potassium vegetables.

How to leach vegetables.

For Potatoes, Sweet Potatoes, Carrots, Beets, and Rutabagas:

1. Peel and place the vegetable in cold water so they won't darken.

2. Slice vegetable 1/8 inch thick.

3. Rinse in warm water for a few seconds.

4. Soak for a minimum of two hours in warm water. Use ten times the amount of water to the amount of vegetables. If soaking longer, change the water every four hours.

5. Rinse under warm water again for a few seconds.

6. Cook vegetable with five times the amount of water to the amount of vegetable.

For Squash, Mushrooms, Cauliflower, and Frozen Greens:

1. Allow frozen vegetable to thaw to room temperature and drain.

2. Rinse fresh or frozen vegetables in warm water for a few seconds.

3. Soak for a minimum of two hours in warm water. Use ten times the amount of water to the amount of vegetables. If soaking longer, change the water every four hours.

4. Rinse under warm water again for a few seconds.

5. Cook the usual way, but with five times the amount of water to the amount of vegetable.

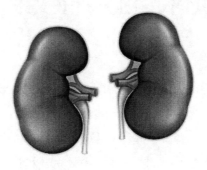

CHAPTER 8

STEP 5 MANAGE YOUR PHOSPHORUS

Phosphorus is a mineral found in your bones. Along with calcium, phosphorus is needed for building healthy strong bones, as well as keeping other parts of your body healthy.

Normal working kidneys can remove extra phosphorus in your blood. With CKD your kidneys may not be as efficient in removing phosphorus very well. Higher phosphorus levels can cause damage to your body. Extra phosphorus causes body changes that pull calcium out of your bones, making them weak.

DO YOU NEED PHOSPHORUS RESTRICTION?

It is not common to see elevated phosphorus level in the early stages of CKD. In stage 4 some patients may need to have more focus in their diet on reducing phosphorus. For most of my patients in the earlier stages of CKD, I ask to stop drinking Coke and Pepsi and to be wary of processed foods where phosphorus is added in the manufacturing process. Read labels and steer away from processed foods. Many natural foods also contain phosphorus but it is not well absorbed so generally we don't worry about it as much.

In some cases, if diet alone cannot control your phosphorus levels your physician may prescribe medication that absorbs the phosphorus in the gastrointestinal track and prevents its absorption.

These are called phosphorus binders. Your doctor may prescribe Renvela, Phos Lo or a generic calcium acetate, Fosrenol or a form of calcium carbonate. Some of these are over the counter but please don't take them until our doctor prescribes it.

Here are some guidelines if you have been told to "watch you phosphorus".

Instead of these higher phosphorus foods:	Choose these lower phosphorus foods:
Milk, pudding or yogurt	Rice milk, almond milk, nondairy creamer, soy milk
Cream soup made with milk	Broth-based soup made with water
Hard cheese	Cream cheese

Instead of these higher phosphorus foods:	Choose these lower phosphorus foods:
Ice cream or frozen yogurt	Sherbet or frozen fruit pops
Fast food chicken	Plain salads or higher quality poultry
Quick breads, biscuits, cornbread, muffins, pancakes or waffles	
Refined dinner rolls, bagels, English muffins or croissants	
Dried peas, beans or lentils	Asparagus, green beans, wax beans, broccoli, beets, cabbage, carrots, cucumbers, peppers, lettuce, onions, tomatoes, spinach or summer squash
Organ meats	poultry or fish
Peanuts	Popcorn
Chocolate	Hard candy or gumdrops
Cola soft drinks	Green or black iced tea made from tea bags. Water Lemon-lime soda, ginger ale or root beer

Even if you don't have a phosphorus problem, these foods cannot be healthy for you so start reading the labels and eliminating them.

Convenience foods, ready to eat and processed foods frequently contain phosphorus additives. Read ingredient labels to find phosphorus additives such as:

Dicalcium phosphate

Disodium phosphate

Monocalcium phosphate

Monosodium phosphate

Potassium tripolyphosphate

Pyrophosphate

Sodium acid pyrophosphate

Sodium aluminum phosphate

Sodium hexametaphosphate

Sodium phosphate

Sodium triphosphate

Tetrasodium pyrophosphate

Tricalcium phosphate

Trisodium triphosphateSource

Source: National Institutes of Health/National Institute of Diabetes and Digestive and Kidney Diseases

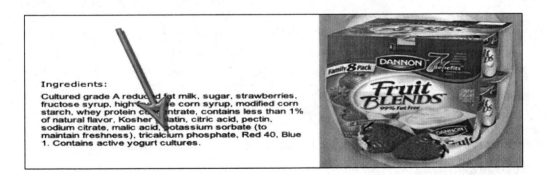

Whole grains: To eat or not to eat?

For many years whole grains have been restricted from the CKD diet. The reason is that they are higher in phosphorus than their less healthy processed flour alternatives. Dietitians have been telling CKD patients for years "no wheat bread, eat white bread instead". This has changed due to research that shows the phosphorus in whole grains is bound to phytates. As mammals we can't break the phytate bond so very little of the phosphorus is actually absorbed. If you prefer whole grain bread and whole grain pasta then consider it perfectly ok to have. Legumes such as beans, lentils are on the be careful list not due to phosphorus but due to the high quantity of potassium. The phosphorus in legumes is also bound to phytates.

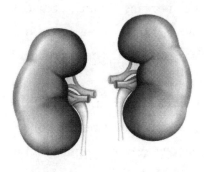

CHAPTER 9

STEP 6 MANAGE YOUR ANEMIA

Anemia is a condition in which the blood does not contain enough red blood cells. These cells are important because they carry oxygen throughout the body. A person who is anemic will feel tired and look pale. Healthy kidneys make the hormone EPO, which stimulates the bones to make red blood cells. Diseased kidneys may not make enough EPO. A person with CKD may need to take injections of EPO

Anemia in Kidney Disease

What is anemia?

A person whose blood is low in red blood cells has anemia. Red blood cells carry oxygen to tissues and organs throughout the body and enable them to use the energy from food.

Without oxygen, these tissues and organs— particularly the heart and brain—may not do their jobs as well as they should. For this reason, a person who has anemia may tire easily and look pale. Anemia may also contribute to heart problems.

Anemia is common in people with kidney disease. Healthy kidneys produce a hormone called erythropoietin, or EPO, which stimulates the bone marrow to produce the proper number of red blood cells needed to carry oxygen to vital organs. Diseased kidneys, however, often don't make enough EPO. As a result, the bone marrow makes fewer red blood cells. In addition low levels of iron and folic acid also contribute to the inefficient production of red blood cells.

What are the laboratory tests for anemia?

A complete blood count (CBC), a laboratory test performed on a sample of blood, includes a determination of a person's hematocrit, the percentage of the blood that consists of red blood cells. The CBC also measures the amount of hemoglobin in the blood. The range of normal hematocrit and hemoglobin in women who have a period is slightly lower than for healthy men and healthy women who have stopped having periods (postmenopausal). The hemoglobin is usually about one-third the value of the hematocrit.

When does anemia begin?

Anemia may begin to develop in the early stages of kidney disease, when you still have 20 percent to 50 percent of your normal kidney function. This partial loss of kidney function is often called chronic renal insufficiency.

How is anemia diagnosed?

If a person has lost at least half of normal kidney function and has a low hematocrit, the most likely cause of anemia is decreased EPO production. The estimate of kidney function, also called the glomerular filtration rate, is based on a blood test that measures creatinine. Experts recommend that doctors begin a detailed evaluation of anemia in men and post-menopausal women on dialysis when the hematocrit falls below 37 percent. For women of childbearing age, evaluation should begin when the hematocrit falls below 33 percent. The evaluation will include tests for iron deficiency and blood loss in the stool to be certain there are no other reasons for the anemia.

How is anemia treated? EPO

If no other cause for anemia is found, it can be treated with a genetically engineered form of EPO. Currently the commercial for of EPO that is used in CKD in called Procrit. It is given by a subcutaneous (under the skin) injection. EPO takes about 2 weeks to start the blood making process in your bone marrow. Many patients feel noticeably better about 2 weeks after their EPO shot.

Iron

Many people with kidney disease need both EPO and iron supplements to raise their hematocrit to a satisfactory level. If a person's iron levels are too low, EPO won't help and that person will continue to experience the effects of anemia. Your physician may recommend iron supplements. Many iron preparations irritate the stomach, can cause constipation or diarrhea. Let your doctor know if you are unable to tolerate your iron supplement and another type may be more suitable for you. If you are unable to tolerate iron orally some doctors will refer you for an iron infusion.

In addition to measuring hematocrit and hemoglobin, the CBC test will include two other measurements to show whether a person has enough iron.

- The ferritin level indicates the amount of iron stored in the body. The ferritin score should be no less than 100 micrograms per liter (mcg/L) and no more than 800 mcg/L.

- TSAT stands for transferrin saturation; a score that indicates how much iron is available to make red blood cells. The TSAT score should be between 20 and 50 percent.

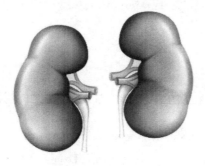

CHAPTER 10

STEP 7 MANAGE YOUR CHOLESTEROL AND START AN EXERCISE PROGRAM

Cholesterol. Another problem that may be associated with kidney failure is high cholesterol. High levels of cholesterol in the blood may result from a high-fat diet.

What is cholesterol?

Cholesterol is a fat-like substance that the body uses to make hormones and cell walls. Cells in the liver make all the cholesterol our body needs.

The body does NOT need the extra cholesterol we get in the foods we eat, which is called dietary cholesterol.

Eating foods high in cholesterol, saturated fat, and trans fats can raise levels of cholesterol in the blood.

What factors tend to raise cholesterol?

Several factors raise blood cholesterol. Some we have no control over, like our genetic make-up and aging bodies. But many we do have control over.

A major controllable factor that raises blood cholesterol levels is a diet high in:

Saturated fats (such as butter, palm oil, coconut oil, meat fats, and milk fats, trans fats (such as margarine, vegetable shortening, and partially hydrogenated oils)

Cholesterol (found ONLY in animal products such as meat and cheese, not plant based foods)

Other controllable factors that raise cholesterol levels include:

> Excessive meal size
>
> Fasting
>
> High fructose corn syrup and sucrose (table sugar)
>
> Weight gain and excess body fat (BMI, or body mass index, greater than 25) Medications (such as diuretics and beta blockers)
>
> Uncontrolled diabetes, hypothyroidism, and other metabolic conditions
>
> Stress

What factors tend to lower LDL
"bad" cholesterol and total cholesterol?

You can lower your LDL and total cholesterol by:

- Eating more fiber (especially soluble fiber from beans, oats, barley, fruits, and vegetables)

- Eating polyunsaturated fatty acids in moderate portions (In large amounts, they promote weight gain and may impair immune function.)

- Eating frequent, smaller meals (grazing) Eating vegetable proteins (such as tofu and beans) in place of meat

- Gradual weight loss

- Eating phytochemicals (i.e., plant sterols) Taking cholesterol-lowering medications

What is HDL cholesterol?

HDL cholesterol is commonly called the "good" cholesterol because it tends to pick up bad cholesterol particles from the blood and artery walls and return them to the liver for disposal. Think of HDL particles as your "garbage workers." HDL garbage workers do a great job of clearing the body of LDL "trash."

How can I raise my HDL "good" cholesterol?

You can raise your HDLs by:

- Exercising – the equivalent of walking 15 to 18 miles per week. Keep in mind, that it takes months of walking, not days, to raise HDL.

- Losing weight (and keeping it off) Quitting smoking

- Medications (after trying lifestyle changes)

- Alcohol (moderation, with doctors permission)

Some people in addition to having high cholesterol also have high triglycerides. This is common in people diagnosed with diabetes.

What is a triglyceride?

A triglyceride is a type of fat. Most of the fats in food are triglycerides. You also have triglycerides in your blood and stored as fat in your body. When you have high levels of triglycerides in blood, you have too much fat circulating in your blood. And you may be at a greater risk for heart disease than if your blood triglyceride levels were low.

The food you eat affects your blood level of triglycerides, so you need to stop eating 14 hours before getting your triglycerides measured. The desired range for triglycerides is between 100 and 150 milligrams per deciliter (mg/dl).

Some people may have extreme levels (1000 or above), but your triglyceride level may be too high if it's above 160 mg/dl, depending on what other risk factors you have for heart disease.

Reasons to Change Your Diet

Your weight can affect your blood triglyceride level. If you are obese (more than 20% above your ideal body weight) or just overweight, you may be able to lower your blood triglycerides by losing weight

Eating a diet low in fat, especially saturated fat, may also help you lower your blood triglyceride level. Use olive oil in cooking and in salad dressing as much as possible

Exercise, in addition to helping with weight loss may also help lower triglyceride levels.

Too many carbohydrates in your diet may also increase your blood triglycerides. You need carbohydrates in your diet, especially the "complex" carbohydrates like bread, rice, potatoes, corn and other starchy vegetables. But should limit "simple" carbohydrates like sugar, candy, honey, and jelly and other items, which may contain excess sugar.

Following The Diet

1. Control calories to reach and maintain your ideal weight

2. Eat low-fat foods instead of high-fat foods. This can help you lose weight, too.

3. These foods are lower in fat. Eat more of these:

   - peas, *dried beans, and *lentils
   - whole grain breads, cereals and pasta
   - egg whites
   - skim and nonfat dry milk

- cheese made with skim or part-skim milk, such as mozzarella, parmesan, farmers', ricotta, or pot cheese

- *low-fat cottage cheese

- *low-fat yogurt

- fish

- poultry without the skin

- lean cuts of meat, such as round, sirloin, rump, and flank (limit to once per week or less due to CKD)

  * considered high in potassium

4. Select olive oil, a monosaturated fat whenever possible.

   If olive oil does not go in your recipe then the second best fat is a unsaturated fat:

- canola oil

- safflower oil

- soybean oil

- sunflower oil

- peanut oil

- margarines made with these oils

- mayonnaise

- almonds

- cashews

- pecans

- peanuts

- peanut butter

- walnuts

- pine nuts

- sunflower seeds

- pumpkin seeds

5. Avoid sugar and other high-sugar foods. This will decrease carbohydrates without decreasing other nutrients. Sugar in your food goes rapidly to your blood. When there is excess sugar in your blood, your liver may use it to make more triglycerides. Sugar also contains calories without other important nutrients.

Eat less of these:

- sugar, brown sugar, powdered sugar, jam, jelly, preserves, honey, syrup, molasses, pies, candy, cakes, cookies, frosting, pastries, colas, soft drinks, , punches, fruit drinks, and regular gelatin

6. Avoid alcohol. Alcohol, will increase blood triglycerides even more than sugar. In addition, alcohol is high in calories and low in nutrients. Ask for sparkling water, or a diet soft drink instead of an alcoholic beverage.

Suggestions for Planning and Preparing Meals

*Bake, broil, or roast meats instead of frying.

*Remove any visible fat from meats and the skin from poultry before cooking.

*Add spices, herbs, lemon juice or vinegar to vegetables instead of rich sauces or gravies.

*Use a non-stick skillet without fat and use no-stick sprays.

*Cool and refrigerate stews and broth. Then remove the hardened fat before serving.

*Serve more fish.

*Use less butter, margarine and other high-fat spreads on bread or vegetables. Use olive oil

*Use skim or reconstituted non-fat dry milk for cooking.

*Cook with low-fat cheeses.

*Substitute low-fat yogurt or cottage cheese for all or part of the sour cream in recipes for sauces, dips or congealed salads.

*Choose fresh fruits for dessert--they are naturally low in fat--instead of high-fat foods such as pies or cakes.

When Dining Out

*Select clear rather than cream soups.

*Ask that dressings and gravies be served on the side. Then use less of them.

*Order foods that are baked, broiled, poached, steamed, stir-fried, or roasted.

*Drink sparkling water, unsweetened tea or coffee

In summary: I hope you are not feeling confused because you have heard this throughout the book: Weight loss, if indicated, use olive oil primarily, avoid sweets and baked goodies, and limit fried foods. Eat more fruits, vegetables, grains, fish and poultry. Add exercise to your life.

Exercise

Exercise is a readily accessible, safe, and inexpensive anti-inflammatory medicine. Inflammation is the body's natural means of stimulating healing,

Exercise signals the release of molecules that stimulate a unique healing response that couples both inflammatory and anti-inflammatory mechanisms to repair, regenerate, and grow stronger tissue

Every time the body moves, muscles release signaling molecules that communicate to the rest of the body. The endocrine properties of muscle, like fat, have been confirmed. In the case of muscle, compounds called myokines are released in response to voluntary contraction. These myokines give instructions to the body about how to function, and they hold the key to controlling chronic inflammation

Now that you are convinced that you should exercise, how should you start?

If you're not sure about becoming active or boosting your level of physical activity because you're afraid of getting hurt, the good news is that **moderate-intensity aerobic activity**, like brisk walking, is generally **safe for most people**.

Start slowly. Cardiac events, such as a heart attack, are rare during physical activity. But the risk does go up when you suddenly become much more active than usual. For example, you can put yourself at risk if you don't usually get much physical activity and then all of a sudden do vigorous-intensity aerobic activity, like shoveling snow. That's why it's important to start slowly and gradually increase your level of activity.

If you have a chronic health condition such as arthritis, diabetes, or heart disease, talk with your doctor to find out if your condition limits, in any way, your ability to be active.

Then, work with your doctor to come up with a physical activity plan that matches your abilities. If your condition stops you from meeting the minimum Guidelines, try to do as much as you can. What's important is that you avoid being inactive. Even 60 minutes a week of moderate-intensity aerobic activity is good for you.

The bottom line is – the health benefits of physical activity far outweigh the risks of getting hurt. Set your goal for 30 minutes of activity daily with two of those days using weights or some other type of resistance exercise. If you have not been active 60 minutes per day does sound impossible. Start slowly with even 10 minutes per day; build up gradually until you are at 30 minutes of daily exercise. Do not over exert yourself; you should always be able to carry on a conversation.

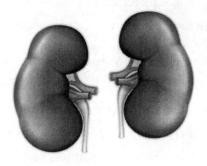

CHAPTER 11

STEP 8 BE AWARE OF MEDICAL TESTING

USE OF NSAIDS AND TOXIC HERBALS

The Society for Cardiovascular Angiography and Interventions (SCAI) has released recommendations for the prevention of contrast-induced nephropathy (CIN) - potentially fatal kidney damage that can occur when a special dye is injected during certain cardiovascular procedures.

Contrast dye is essential for many diagnostic and interventional cardiovascular procedures because it enables doctors to visualize blocked blood

Recommendations given to physicians:

1. Make sure patients are adequately hydrated before, during, and after the procedure. Hydration is very important in preventing CIN.

2. Address with patients whether to discontinue the use of non-steroidal anti-inflammatory (NSAID) agents 24-48 hours before a procedure. Medications such as ibuprofen and Naprosyn are known as NSAIDs and are usually taken for aches and pains associated with arthritis, headache, back injury, and other ailments. These medications can potentially cause a kidney problem by decreasing blood flow to the kidneys. Because contrast dyes can also decrease kidney blood flow, the two agents should not be given concurrently.

3. In patients at increased risk for CIN, use contrast agents with lower osmolality, and in the smallest possible quantities. Contrast agents with lower osmolality are less dense and, therefore, less likely to interfere with blood flow to the kidneys.

4. Monitor patients at increased risk for CIN very closely for up to 48 hours after a procedure that involved the use of contrast dye. Physicians and nurses should be on the lookout for any signs of kidney failure. During this period, the serum creatinine test is useful for monitoring kidney function. In addition, patients should not resume taking NSAIDs until their kidney function has returned to normal.

Persons with kidney disease should avoid contrast dyes that contain iodine, if possible. These dyes are removed through the kidneys and can worsen kidney function.

Certain imaging tests use these types of dyes. If they must be used, fluids should be given through a vein for several hours before the test. This allows for rapid removal of the dyes from the body.

NON STEROIDAL
ANTI INFLAMAATORY DRUGS

Commonly used nonsteroidal anti-inflammatory drugs (NSAIDs), including ibuprofen, naproxen, and prescription COX-2 inhibitors such as celecoxib (Celebrex), may injure the weakened kidney. They diminish the blood flow to the kidneys. If your kidney function is already decreased the use of these NSAIDS can be potentially harmful.

Here is a list of commonly used NSAIDS in the United States.

celecoxib	(Celebrex) diclofenac
(Voltaren) diflunisal	(Dolobid) etodolac
(Lodine) ibuprofen	(Motrin)
indomethacin	(Indocin)
ketoprofen	(Orudis)
ketorolac	(Toradol)
nabumetone	(Relafen)
naproxen	(Aleve, Naprosyn)
oxaprozin	(Daypro)
piroxicam	(Feldene)
salsalate	(Amigesic)
sulindac	(Clinoril)
tolmetin	(Tolectin)

Many Nephrologists recommend the use of Tylenol as a routine painkiller. Remember that Tylenol and alcohol is a harmful combination for your liver.

Ask your doctor what he recommends for you and don't take any medication without your doctor' approval.

National Institute of Health's (NIH) List of Harmful and Toxic Herbs

Herbals are often marketed as having healing properties; the FDA markets them as a food supplement therefore not subjected to the rigorous screening for safety and efficacy. People with decreased kidney function are especially at risk whey they try a substance which may be eliminated by the kidneys but whose safety record has not been established. Recently the National Institute of Health put out a comprehensive list of herbs that should be avoided:

Herbs that may be **toxic** to the kidneys:

> Artemisia, Absinthium (wormwood plant)
>
> Autumn crocus,
>
> Chuifong tuokuw (Black Pearl),
>
> Horse chestnut,
>
> Periwinkle,
>
> Sassafras,
>
> Tung shueh,
>
> Vanda cordifolia

Herbs that may be **harmful** in chronic kidney disease:

Alfalfa,

Aloe,

Bayberry,

Blue Cohosh,

Broom,

Coltsfoot,

Buckthorn,

Capsicum

Cascara,

Dandelion,

Ginger,

Ginseng,

Horsetail,

Licorice,

Mate,

Nettle,

Noni Juice,

Panax,

Senna,

Vervain

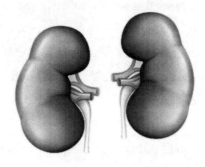

CHAPTER 12

STEP 9 VIT D, ANTI-INFLAMATORY AND ANTIOXIDATS

Vitamin D

Increasingly, vitamin D insufficiency is being seen as a health concern in many individuals but especially those with chronic kidney disease. We obtain Vitamin D from sunlight and convert it in the kidney to a usable form. Due to limited time spent outdoors and the kidney inability to convert the Vitamin D to its active form, leads many patients with CKD to be vitamin D deficient.

Decreased Vitamin D can lead to increased risk of osteoporosis, muscle weakness, falls, fractures and a weakened immune system.

Vitamin D status is most accurately determined by direct measurement of serum 25-OH-Groups at greatest risk of vitamin D insufficiency include young children and women, particularly those in middle and advanced ages, and inactive elderly people in general. Current recommendations indicate a daily vitamin D intake of 400-600 IU and a calcium intake of 1000-1200 mg/dl, but some patients may require even higher intake of vitamin D to achieve desirable serum vitamin D concentrations. If a Vitamin D deficiency is diagnosed your doctor may recommend 2000 iu of Vitamin D daily or higher doses taken weekly.

Maintenance of adequate vitamin D status is also important in patients with chronic kidney disease (CKD). Vitamin D deficiency develops as early as stage 3 of CKD factors. In patients with CKD, Vit D (25-OH-D) levels should be maintained at greater than 30 ng/ml. Your doctor will measure your vitamin D levels to see if you are above 30 ng/ml.

Antioxidants and Anti-inflammatory

The beneficial health effects of olive oil are due to both its high content of monounsaturated fatty acids and its high content of antioxidative and anti-inflammatory substances. Research now shows that many of olive oil's health benefits may actually come from the more than 30 plant compounds it contains.

These compounds' antioxidant and anti-inflammatory effects are due to a naturally occurring chemical found in extra-virgin olive oils is a non-steroidal anti-inflammatory agent. Named oleocanthal by the researchers, the compound inhibits activity of cyclooxygenase (COX) enzymes, a pharmacological action shared by ibuprofen.

The finding is significant because inflammation increasingly is believed to play a key role in a variety of chronic diseases. "Some of the health-related effects of the Mediterranean diet may be due to the natural anti-COX activity of oleocanthal from premium olive oils

Researchers believe components of olive oil such as flavonoids, squalenecontain the antioxidants hydroxytyrosol, oleuropein, and tyrosol found in the extra-virgin olive oil helped patients to control blood pressure levels. Scientists conclude that a diet lower in total fat and saturated fat and a diet that contains higher amounts of MUFA can lower blood pressure levels.

Which type of olive oil to purchase?

All types of olive oil provide the monounsaturated fat linked with health benefits, but to get the highest levels of the protective plant compounds, choose "extra virgin" or "virgin" oil, the least processed forms. Store it away from light and heat to maintain phytochemical content.

Hydroxytyrosol and **tyrosol** are some of the many **phenol compounds** in olive oil that contribute to bitter taste, astringency, and resistance to oxidation. They are now being played up in the press as a desirable health component of olive oil. The flavonoid polyphenols in olive oil are natural anti-oxidants that have been shown to have a host of beneficial effects from healing sunburn to lowering cholesterol, blood pressure, and risk of coronary disease. There are as many as 5 mg of antioxidant polyphenols in every 10 grams of olive oil. Many other nut and seed oils have no polyphenols. Phenol content is determined by **olive variety; time of picking, oil processing method**, whether the oil is refined and the length of time the oil has been **stored**.

Variety - Specific types of olives, such as the Tuscan varieties, will have higher polyphenol values. These oils are valuable in that when blended with low polyphenol oil they will extend the shelf life by preventing rancidity.

Processing method - Much is made of how the type of olive oil machinery will affect the flavor of extra virgin oil but in reality if used properly it has only a small influence. **Extra virgin olive oil** is made the same way with the same machinery in the US as in Italy. Only a tiny percent of the oil sold in the US is made in the US and is mostly artisanal extra virgin oil, which is **high** in phenols.

Most of the olive oil consumed in the US comes from Spain and Italy, and is usually refined. These mass-market oils are generally refined and low in phenols.

Refining takes olive oil which has already been made but which is old, rancid, was made from diseased olives or has some other sort of defect and makes it palatable. This is done by filtering, charcoal treatment, heating, and chemical treatment to adjust acidity. Refined oils are lower in tyrosol and other phenols. According to Wayne Emmons at Intertech, **Extra Virgin Olive oil** typically has **50-80 ppm** polyphenols while **refined oil** has only **5 ppm**.

Storage - As oil sits in storage tanks or the bottle, the polyphenols will slowly be oxidized and used up. If you want oil with more polyphenols, buy one that displays a date guaranteeing that it is fresh and that has been stored properly.

Hydroxytyrosol and other phenols are not used in any legal definition so you can only make generalizations to how many there are in various types of oil. Oils labeled as "lite" or "light" refer to flavor, not caloric content, as all vegetable oils have the same amount of calories. Theoretically "light" could refer to excellent extra virgin oil made from olives picked late in the year but usually it signifies a flavorless low quality (refined) oil from Italy or Spain.

If you want an oil high in polyphenols, pick one that is guaranteed to be extra virgin (has the COOC seal if produced in the US), is from the current harvest season and that has been properly stored. Some varieties have high polyphenols; Frantoio, Lucca, etc. Look for US oils made from these varieties or look in a quality store or deli for a high quality extra virgin oil made with care and well labeled.

Omega-3 fatty acids

A diet rich in Omega 3 fatty acids has been shown to decrease inflammation, which may reduce your risk for developing chronic disease and inflammatory conditions such as cardiovascular disease, diabetes and CKD. Our diets tend to be higher in Omega 6 fatty acids – high amounts found in meats, dairy, eggs and some vegetable oils – and lower in omega 3's. This imbalance may increase your risk for inflammation. To create a better fatty acid balance, start incorporating more omega 3 fatty acids into your diet by increasing cold water fish, flax, walnuts, pumpkin seeds and soybeans, and decreasing Omega 6 foods. Finding a balance with these nutrients is an important step in decreasing your risk for developing chronic disease. Supplementing with Omega 3 is also recommended in the following quantities.

1.8 g/day of EPA + 1.2 g/day of DHA) for two years significantly slowed declines in renal function.

Supplement Facts
Serving Size 1 Soft Gelatin Capsule

Amount Per Serving	
Calories: 10	Calories From Fat: 10
	Amount
Total Fat	1 g
Polyunsaturated Fat	0.5 g
Vitamin E (d-alpha tocopherol)	1.1 iu
Fish Oil	1000 mg
EPA (eicosapentaenoic acid from fish oil)	**680 mg**
DHA (Docosahexaenoic Acid)	**520 mg**

**Percent Daily Values are based on a 2,000 calorie diet. *Daily Value n established

Read the label and determine the actual amount of EPA and DHA that is provided. You may have to take 2 to 3 capsules to get the required amount. With the above label 2 capsules will provide 1,360mg or 1.36 gm or EPA and 1,040 mg or 1.0 gm of DHA which is close enough to the recommendations.

TEA

If you are looking for a healthy beverage to drink, look no further than tea.

Tea contains Vitamins A, C, and E, as well as healthy compounds called Flavonoids. The flavonoid in tea, called polyphenols, are antioxidants that give tea, all its healthy benefits. One subgroup of polyphenols, called catechins, is abundant in tea - Catechins were discovered in the '70s, when scientists were trying to figure out why people in Japan's Shizuoka Prefecture - a major tea growing area - had substantially lower rates of cancer than other Japanese, even when they were heavy smokers. One specific catechin, epigallocatechin gallate (EGCg), is found in no other plant other than tea, and it's one of the most potent antioxidants

Tea, whether black or green, caffeinated or decaffeinated (herbal teas don't count), has spectacular antioxidant capabilities owing to large amounts of substances called flavonoids. In addition to preventing oxidation, flavonoids may have an anticlotting effect.

Bag it. When Consumer Reports tested the antioxidant punch of 15 brewed, bottled, and instant teas, it found most teas brewed from tea bags scored highest in antioxidant content. In fact, the magazine reported, "Brewed tea appears to have more antioxidant action than almost any whole fruit or vegetable -- and more than most commercial fruit or vegetable juices, too." But iced teas from mixes and bottle are a decent second choice; they contain a "good deal" of antioxidants, according to the magazine. Just watch the sugar content.

Dunk the bag. Continuously dunking the tea bag, as the tea steeps seems to release far more antioxidant compounds than simply dropping it in and leaving it there.

Add lemon. One study found that the addition of lemon to plain tea increased its antioxidant benefits. That makes sense, since lemon itself contains antioxidants.

Brew a batch. To make a day's supply of iced tea, bring 20 ounces of water to a boil, and then remove from the heat. Drop in three tea bags, cover, and steep for 10 minutes. Remove tea bags and refrigerate.

Try green tea. Because it isn't fermented, green tea has even more antioxidant power than black tea does. It also has less caffeine. And it may provide some protection against certain cancers. Experiment with brands until you find one you like.

Don't let green tea steep for more than a couple of minutes or it may become bitter.

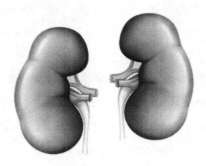

STEP 10 RECENT RESEARCH

Journal of the American Society of Nephrology

Daily supplementation with sodium bicarbonate slows the progression rate of renal failure to end-stage renal disease (ESRD) and improves nutritional status among patients with chronic kidney disease (CKD), according to a randomized, open-label study reported online July 16, 2009 in the *Journal of the American Society of Nephrology*

The study, led by Dr. Magdi Yaqoob, at Royal London Hospital, included 134 patients with advanced CKD and low bicarbonate levels, also called metabolic acidosis.

All patients were randomly assigned to receive either 600 mg oral sodium bicarbonate tablet or placebo.

At the end of the study, the rate of decline in creatinine clearance was significantly slower for those treated with the bicarbonate supplementation compared with the control group

"This is the first randomized, controlled clinical study in which oral sodium bicarbonate supplementation was associated with positive results in both primary and secondary end-points in patients with CKD," the study authors write. In addition, "there was no effect on [blood pressure] or evidence of worsening edema as assessed clinically at every clinic consultation."

The rate of decline in kidney function was greatly reduced- about two-thirds slower than in patients who did not receive the sodium bicarbonate.

"In fact, in patients taking sodium bicarbonate, the rate of decline in kidney function was similar to the normal age- related decline," said Yaqoob.

Patients taking sodium bicarbonate were less likely to develop end-stage renal disease (ESRD) requiring dialysis and also had improvement in several measures of nutritional status.

Although their sodium levels went up, this didn't lead to any problems with increased blood pressure.

Oral sodium bicarbonate supplementation in patients with low plasma HCO_3 – levels slows the rate of decline of renal function and the development of ESRD in patients with advanced stages of CKD," the study authors conclude.

New use for Acthar to treat proteinuria:

Acthar is an FDA-approved prescription treatment that helps to lower protein in people with excess urinary protein. This condition is called proteinuria in nephrotic syndrome. Acthar contains the hormone ACTH, which stands for adrenocorticotropic hormone. Acthar is a highly purified preparation of ACTH in gelatin.

Acthar binds to specific receptors in the body (often called melanocortin "receptors" or "MCRs" by healthcare professionals). There are 5 different types of these receptors throughout the body, and Acthar binds to all 5 of them. Some of these MCR receptors are found in the adrenal cortex. This is the outer portion of the adrenal gland found on the top of each of your kidneys.

STUDY SUGGESTS A LITTLE WINE MAY BE GOOD FOR YOUR KIDNEYS

National Kidney Foundation Meetings Spring 2014
Moderate wine consumption could help keep the kidneys healthy, and may protect the heart in patients who already have kidney disease, according to new findings

Tapan Mehta, MD, of the University of Colorado-Denver, and his colleagues found that people who drank less than one glass of wine a day had a 37 percent lower prevalence of chronic kidney disease than those who drank no wine at all. Among study participants who had chronic kidney disease, those who drank less than a glass of wine daily were 29 percent less likely to have cardiovascular disease than non-wine drinkers.

"Similar to previous studies showing that moderate wine consumption appears to impart some health benefit by lowering the risk of heart disease and diabetes, this study suggests an association between moderate wine consumption (< 1 glass/day) and lower rates of chronic kidney disease."

Moderation is the key for kidney patients when it comes to alcohol consumption, with a few caveats, "Excess alcohol consumption has definitely been shown to have negative effects on kidney function."

Vegetarian Diets Compared to Meat Dietary Protein l ed to decreased blood phosphorus levels.

Clinical Journal of American Society of Nephrology

Subjects with chronic kidney disease who had elevated phosphorus and PTH levels were followed .

One group ate a traditional American diet, the other group followed a vegetarian diet. During the study it was found that the vegetarian diets promoted a drop in serum phosphorus and PTH while the traditional American diet had no decrease in phosphorus levels.

NEW DRUG FOR FSGS

Possible new drug for Focal Segmental Glomerular Sclerosis a drug approved for the treatment of rheumatoid arthritis may also turn out to be the first targeted therapy for one of the most common forms of kidney disease. A team led by researchers at Harvard-affiliated Massachusetts General Hospital (MGH) is reporting that treatment with abatacept (Orencia) appeared to halt the course of focal segmental glomerulosclerosis (FSGS) in five patients, preventing four from losing transplanted kidneys and achieving disease remission in the fifth. The report was issued online in the New England Journal of Medicine (NEJM).

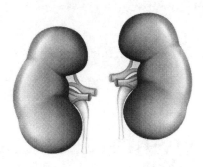

LOW OXALATE DIET

For prevention of kidney stones or reduction of urine oxalate and citrate

Kidney stones are pieces of stone like material that form on the walls of the kidney. They are caused by a buildup of minerals in the urine.

Step 1. Plan your diet to stay within approximately 40 – 50 mg of oxalate per day.

Step 2 HYDRATE people who are likely to develop kidney stones should drink 8-13 cups of fluid per day. Your urine should be pale yellow to indicate adequate hydration.

Step 3 Avoid Vitamin C supplementation or beverages with Vitamin C added

Step 4 Do not take any calcium supplements, foods with calcium such as dairy is OK

Step 5 Follow recommended protein allowance

Step 6 Use non-steroidal anti-inflammatory medicines with caution and not for chronic use.

FOOD, WHICH CAN CAUSE A HIGH URINARY OXALATE CONTENT:

- Spinach, rhubarb, beets (both the root and the greens), nuts and nut butters, chocolate and cocoa, green and black tea, wheat bran (in high amounts), soybeans and foods made from soy, and strawberries.

- Other foods commonly held to contain high oxalate, such as cola beverages and coffee, do not actually contain much oxalate. Stone formers may consume these beverages in moderation as part of an overall healthy diet.

If you absorb too much oxalate from the foods in your diet, your risk for calcium oxalate stones increases dramatically. How does oxalate absorption get too high?

- HIGH OXALATE ABSORBTION DUE TO CONSUMING IT WITH FAT. Some individuals absorb too much oxalate because: (a) their dietary fat intake is too high; Oxalate is fat-soluble, so reducing the fat you eat, especially saturated fat, may reduce the amount of oxalate you absorb. Saturated fat is fat found in animal protein, full fat dairy and butter

- HIGH Oxalate DUE TO INADEQUATE CALCIUM INTAKE absorption is dramatically decreased with an appropriate amount of calcium consumed at meal times, when you are most likely to consume plant foods that contain oxalate. Thus, individuals who don't require a severe oxalate restriction can still eat those healthy foods if they take care to have a small glass of milk or other calcium-rich food at every meal. When the oxalate and the calcium are present in the GI tract at the same time, they bind together and neither is absorbed.

Other strategies that may be suggested to reduce urinary oxalate excretion include vitamin B6 (also known as pyridoxine) in high doses and probiotic therapy. Vitamin B6, which is available over the counter in 25- or 50-mg tablets, may reduce the amount of oxalate your body produces. Subsequent analysis of your 24-hour urine will determine if this therapy is successful. Probiotic therapy with bacteria of the oxalobacter and possibly lactic acid type may be useful to reduce urinary oxalate; studies are pending. Talk with your physician about it.

Summary

HYDRATE people who are likely to develop kidney stones should drink 8-13 cups of fluid per day.

Avoid Vitamin C supplementation or beverages with Vitamin C added

Check with your doctor prior to taking calcium supplements, foods with calcium such as dairy is OK and beneficial with meals.

Follow recommended protein allowance this will also reduce your intake of saturated fat.

Use non steroidal anti inflammatory medicine with caution and not for chronic use

Sample menu

Breakfast

Cheese omlette

Oat bran bread toasted with margarine, jam ½ glass skim milk or yogurt

Or

Kellogg's Complete Oat Bran Flakes

Milk

½ c blueberries

coffee

Lunch

Grilled chicken on

Iceberg or romaine lettuce salad, cucumbers, onions, cauliflower, green pepper, mushrooms, 2 tomato slices, low fat cheese

Olive oil and vinegar dressing

Grapes

water

Snack

Fruit yogurt

Dinner

Grilled Cod

Squash and zucchini medley

White rice

Red wine

Greek yogurt for dessert

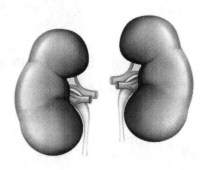

CHAPTER 15

CONCLUSION

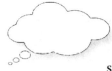 I know I packed a lot of information in a small space, and it may take you a day or two to digest it and formulate a plan. Your action plan should look like this.

1. Control your blood pressure

2. Control your blood sugar

3. Calculate your protein needs and adjust your portions accordingly

4. Select fruits and vegetables from the low and moderate potassium group

5. Avoid Coke, Pepsi and processed foods

6. Change to using olive oil exclusively

7. Stop using non-steroidal medications and check with your doctor prior to having medical testing done.

8. Step up your use of antioxidants by drinking tea, eating a variety of fruit

and vegetables (as allowed) and start supplementing with Vitamin D and Omega 3 Fatty Acids

9. Obtain copies of all your lab tests and plot them on the grid provided in this book. If you see changes ask your doctor.

10. Start an exercise plan

These are all healthy changes that members of your family could join you in following. Many patients have successfully followed this healthy plan and are enjoying full and active lives with fewer health problems. You can do this too! Take charge of your health and your destiny. Your motivation is already showing. You did your research, purchased this book and now take charge of your eating and lifestyle. You may have occasional lapses, don't beat yourself up over it, just make the next choice a healthy choice and move on. With every healthy decision you make you are taking steps to improve your health.

This book is meant to be a companion to my cookbook, Kidney Health Gourmet, Diet Guide and Cookbook. The first cookbook devoted to CKD patients not on dialysis. Each recipe is meticulously analyzed for protein, potassium, phosphorus and sodium (as well as many other nutrients). The recipes were prepared and tested, only the highest rated recipes made it into the book.

There is more dietary information in the book, restaurant guide a beverage and snack guide. I actually compare different types of lettuce and give you potassium information.

Take the guesswork out of your meals and the stress out of your life by preparing healthy meals that you know are safe for your health.

The cookbook can be ordered from www.kidneyhealthgourmet.com or Amazon

If you prefer email me nina@kidneyhealthgourmet.com we can discuss ordering from me directly. If you need help with any of the calculations email me and I can help.

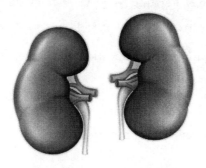

REFERENCES

National Heart Lung and Blood Institute

National Kidney Foundation / Kidney Disease Outcome Initiative

National Kidney Foundation, Council on Renal Nutrition

National Medical Association

Renal Physicians Association Clinical Practice Guidelines

National Diabetes Association

National Kidney Disease Education Program

National Institutes of Health Complementary and Alternative Medicine

The Antioxidant Effect of Tea: Evidence from Human Clinical Trials

The American Society for Nutritional Sciences J. Nutr. 133:3285S-3292S, October 2003

Watkins BA, Hannon K, Ferruzzi M, Li Y. "Dietary PUFA and flavonoids as deterrents for environmental pollutants." J Nutr Biochem. 2009

Mayo Foundation for Medical Education and Research (MFMER) 1998-2009

July 16, 2009 Journal of the American Society of Nephrology Baking soda can slow chronic kidney disease progression.

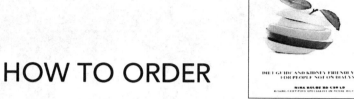

HOW TO ORDER

You may order one or both
books by sending your check or money order to:

Nina Kolbe 215 E. Street SE
Washington, DC 20003
Email: nina@kidneyhealthgourmet.com

❏ I would like to order _____ copy of Kidney Health Gourmet for
$12.99 and $5.00 shipping. Total $17.99

❏ I would like to order ____copy of Avoid Dialysis 10 Step Diet Plan
$12.99 and $ 5.00 shipping. Total $17.99

❏ I would like to order both copies for $30.00 with free shipping

Name _____

Mailing address_____

_____

_____

You can order online on Amazon or
www.kidneyhealthgourmet.com

Questions call 202 390-8044

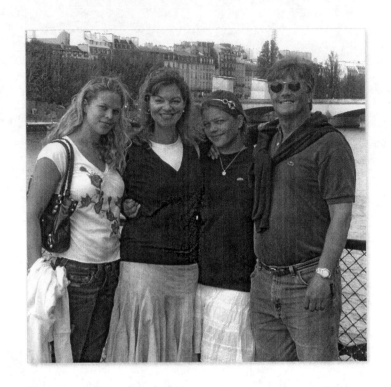

ABOUT THE AUTHOR

Nina Kolbe RD CSR LD has been a practicing dietitian for over 22 years. She has chosen to specialize in kidney disease and became one of the first dietitians in the country to take the board certification exam to earn the title of Certified Renal Specialist. To maintain this certification 75 hours of continuing education must be maintained in the field of kidney disease. This assures the patients that they are receiving the most up to date information from their health professional.

Nina Kolbe maintains a private practice with many physicians in the Washington DC metro area referring to her for nutritional counseling. In addition to a private practice Nina also serves on the medical steering committee board of National Institutes of Health Kidney Disease Education Program, the medical steering committee of the National Kidney Foundation. She has been the chairperson for Council of Renal Nutrition, a Renal Dietitian group for 3 years.

Nina Kolbe has conducted research in the field of renal nutrition. She has presented her research at the National Kidney Foundation's Clinical Meetings. She has been published in the medical journal, Nephrology News & Issues. Is frequently asked to give talks to health professionals in the field on renal nutrition.

This passion and dedication to her profession stems from the belief that early diagnosis, medical and nutritional intervention can delay the progression of kidney disease and depending when treatment is started, avoid dialysis.

CPSIA information can be obtained at www.ICGtesting.com
Printed in the USA
BVOW01s0346290115

385530BV00003B/13/P